FROM *the* HEART

FROM *the* HEART

A Woman's Guide
to Living Well with
Heart Disease

Kathy Kastan,
LCSW, MAEd

President, WomenHeart:
The National Coalition for
Women with Heart Disease

Da Capo
LIFE
LONG

A Member of the
Perseus Books Group

Designed by Timm Bryson
Set in 10.5-point Palatino by the Perseus Books Group

Cataloging-in-Publication data for this book is available from the Library of Congress.

ISBN-13: 978-0-7382-1093-3
ISBN-10: 0-7382-1093-5

Published by Da Capo Press
A Member of the Perseus Books Group
http://www.dacapopress.com

Note: The information in this book is true and complete to the best of our knowledge. This book is intended only as an informative guide for those wishing to know more about health issues. In no way is this book intended to replace, countermand, or conflict with the advice given to you by your own physician. The ultimate decision concerning care should be made between you and your doctor. We strongly recommend you follow his or her advice. Information in this book is general and is offered with no guarantees on the part of the authors or Da Capo Press. The author and publisher disclaim all liability in connection with the use of this book. The names and identifying details of people associated with events described in this book have been changed. Any similarity to actual persons is coincidental.

This book is dedicated to my three wonderful and amazing sons, Benjamin, Nathaniel, and Jonathan, whom I love with all of my heart and soul. Without their computer savvy and emotional support, I doubt this project would ever have gotten off the ground. To my dogs, Millie and Maxie, who give me pet therapy every day. And to Mike, my husband, the love of my life, my best friend and biggest fan—I am truly blessed!

CONTENTS

FOREWORD

From vibrant to vulnerable, from stalwart to shattered, from energetic and in control to emotionally challenged—these are the acute transitions women who sustain a coronary event (a heart attack or a coronary revascularization procedure) experience. Making these transitions, facilitating the recovery process, and not just surviving but thriving—these are the core subjects of Kathy Kastan's *From the Heart: A Woman's Guide to Living Well with Heart Disease.*

As a cardiologist who has provided care for women with heart disease over several decades, I can offer the most advanced medical and surgical therapies, guide preventive and rehabilitative interventions, and counsel and support my patients, but I cannot provide the personal perspective of Kathy Kastan and her interviewees. As a physician with a passion for the benefits of cardiac rehabilitation, I applaud the support for cardiac rehab offered by Kathy and the other heart disease survivors.

Women face so many challenges after a heart event, and Kathy gives straightforward information on a wide range of practical matters. She discusses: How best to take one's heart disease and cardiac symptoms seriously (and to advocate for other women to do so as well) when confronting the challenge of an invisible illness and the frustrations of appearing outwardly healthy but dealing with numerous restrictions. How to avoid being overwhelmed by the myriad lifelong lifestyle changes and multiple medications necessary to reduce coronary risk. How to develop appropriate expectations vis-à-vis family, friends, and coworkers—and to communicate the need for social support versus unwelcome overprotection and emotional smothering. How to transform a woman's traditional role from that of caring for others to that of caring for yourself—and then to perceive yourself not as a victim, but as a victor. How to appreciate that your challenges are not unique but even commonplace, and how to benefit from, to become empowered by, solutions crafted by other women's responses to fear, to guilt, to depression, and the need for diet and exercise.

Physical recovery from a coronary event often comes before emotional recovery. As a first person raconteur, Kathy Kastan and her cosurvivors share the journey back from the loss of self to the rediscovery and renewal that heart patients can ultimately experience. As president of WomenHeart, Kathy and the rest of the organization have performed a great service by facilitating the sharing of information and experiences among women with heart disease, offering reassurance, and suggesting approaches to problem solving at home and in the community—both early in the course of the cardiac illness and well into recovery. This book is a natural offshoot of that process. It shares much-needed information with fellow heart patients. It teaches and coaches by providing examples of how to plan, organize, and assess your cardiac recovery just as you structured your family schedules, your business activities, and your community responsibilities. It also inspires, guiding women through a healthy emotional recovery. As such, it's a very personal and invaluable contribution to the literature on healing women's hearts—and should be spectacularly helpful to women heart patients.

Nanette K. Wenger, MD, MACP, FACC, FAHA

Professor of Medicine (Cardiology),
Emory University School of Medicine
Chief of Cardiology, Grady Memorial Hospital
Consultant, Emory Heart and Vascular Center

INTRODUCTION
A New Beginning: From Nightmare to Daybreak—My Story

Never doubt that a small, group of thoughtful,
committed citizens can change the world.
Indeed, it is the only thing that ever has.
—Margaret Mead

It may be hard to imagine how—in a flash—everything you know can change. How you look at the world. How you think and feel about yourself and your body. How others see you. One minute, you're riding a bike, crossing the street, sitting in a business meeting, or dropping your kids off at school, and then suddenly everything changes. And it changes again. And then again. That's a bit of what my life felt like about six years ago, following a series of unsettling and life-changing events that began with a bike ride with some friends.

During the ride I started having left arm pain. I became short of breath and experienced a pain in my shoulder and back. I felt nauseated, and became pale and light-headed. In fact, these were symptoms I had experienced off and on over the previous eight months while I was running, swimming, or biking. Like most women, I had a lot on my plate. So I just didn't pay much attention to the symptoms—or I attributed them to everything going on in my life instead of what my body was telling me. I thought I was experiencing stresses related to a move the preceding year from Baltimore to Memphis or that maybe my symptoms had something to do with the fact that I'd just turned forty.

The year hadn't been an easy one. I had to close down my psychotherapy practice after fourteen years, find a new house, sell the old one, pack, and help my children adjust to moving from the East Coast to the South. My mother, who lived in California, died at age sixty-one, shortly before the move. The day we buried my mother, my eighty-five-year-old grandma fell and broke her hip and both wrists. I was left with much of the responsibility of dealing with both my mother's estate and my grandmother's incapacity. Like anyone going through so many major changes all at once—a move, leaving a career behind, aiding a disabled grandmother, and adjusting to being a motherless daughter—I found it a stressful and emotionally laden time.

In contrast, once I moved I didn't think life could get any better. I saw myself as a blessed woman—healthy and optimistic. I had three wonderful sons, an intelligent, caring, and successful husband, and a wonderful life full of friends and good times. At thirty-nine, I thought I was invincible and rightly so. I had always been an athlete; I didn't smoke and I ate well. I maintained an average weight and I was fit and active. I involved myself in numerous community activities, rode horses, biked with my friends, swam, ran or walked, and embraced a freedom I had never experienced before in my life. But within a year and what seemed like a blink of an eye, my sense of security, invincibility, and mortality changed forever.

Following the biking episode, my husband, who is a physician, and my friends urged me to see a cardiologist. However, my husband didn't think that what I was experiencing was cardiovascular and told me not to worry.

The first cardiologist diagnosed me with a seemingly benign heart problem called mitral valve prolapse. While I was doing the EKG (electrocardiogram) test on the treadmill, he asked me how I felt and I told him I had tingling down my arm. He said it was probably muscular and connected to my weight lifting. He dismissed me with instructions to drink a lot of water and take antibiotics before each dental visit. He also said he never wanted to see me again because I was the healthiest patient he had ever seen.

The next week, I was in the mountains on vacation, running across a street to post some letters to my sons at camp, when the mild symptoms I'd been having turned into classic, full-blown "Hollywood Heart Attack" symptoms—front to back chest pain, pain radiating down my left arm and into my neck. I was nauseated and sweating profusely, pale, and light-headed. I collapsed on the sidewalk. I'd been drinking a lot of water, just as my cardiologist had advised, and I couldn't imagine why I felt as if I was having a heart attack when the week before he'd told me that I was so healthy. I looked up at the sky and said to myself, "Well, if I am going to die, at least this is one of the most beautiful places on earth." Within about fifteen minutes, I started to feel better, and went back to the hotel and slept for four hours. It never occurred to me to go to the emergency room. But after surviving this incident, my husband and I knew that I needed to get a second opinion.

A new cardiologist confirmed that I had been misdiagnosed. But when he looked at the test results from the echocardiogram that he had performed and the results from the first cardiologist, he was perplexed and had no explanation for my symptoms. He sent me home to exercise to recreate my symptoms—so he could see if they would recur. Those symptoms in the mountains had been very real and I felt as if no one believed me. I was angry and frustrated. It took me four days to get up the courage to try to recreate my symptoms through exercise. Feeling rebellious and angry, I foolishly decided to exercise without anyone around. Within minutes of running on the street, I collapsed again with those same terrifying symptoms that I had had in the mountains. From my cell phone I called my husband, who was angry with me for running without anyone around me. I told him, "Honey, if I am having a heart attack, now is not a good time to yell at me." Of course, he was right. I stupidly had put myself in danger to "show that doctor." After all, to my way of thinking, if the doctor had been that concerned about me, surely he wouldn't have sent me out to exercise. He would have run more tests.

After hearing about my latest episode, the same cardiologist had me run on a treadmill the next day with an echocardiogram and an EKG. Watching the EKG, he got pasty pale and his jaw dropped. Then he left the room to consult with his colleagues. "Kathy," he said when he returned a few minutes later, "I can't believe this, but the results show you have a blockage. I have to catheterize you."

I knew at that instant that my life would change forever. On one hand, I was relieved at the news that my symptoms were real because for months I had thought that maybe I was going crazy. But at that very same moment I was terrified. Over the next eight months I felt like I was on a horrible roller-coaster ride; treatments either failed or caused other complications. Ultimately, I had bypass surgery, a full year after my initial symptoms had begun. That was five years ago.

My experience in the surgical intensive care unit (ICU) following bypass was a nightmare in itself. The nurse who was supposed to care for me was like Nurse Ratched from *One Flew Over the Cuckoo's Nest*. Both the day I came out of surgery and the day after, this nurse didn't take the time, energy, or interest in caring for or supporting me. She was unresponsive to my pain and suffering, and she left me unattended for hours, both when my breathing tube was in right after surgery and the next day when I was in pain. I had complications from the surgery, which added to my physical immobility and helplessness. I couldn't cry out the first day because I had a tube down my throat. The next day I couldn't reach my call light to get someone else to help me out because I was so swollen I couldn't roll over by myself. For two days, all I could do was lie there helplessly and watch the nurse wander in and out of the room for hours, literally ignoring me. This lack of nursing support left me feeling totally demoralized, abandoned, uncomfortable, and scared.

When my family and a friend came in during visiting hours, they found me there sobbing uncontrollably. Not only did I feel humiliated by the nurse, but I was so distraught that I couldn't explain what had happened to me, which was embarrassing as well. No matter how hard I tried to explain it, they didn't understand how that one nurse's blatant disregard had affected me, how vulnerable I was and how frightened.

After eight months of uncertainty and frustration, of dealing with physicians who didn't take me seriously and treatments that didn't work, that one nurse in that one hospital had pushed me over the edge. A year and a half later, I was diagnosed with post-traumatic stress disorder. Ultimately, I went through months of therapy to work through the experience.

Believe it or not, I was still severely ill after bypass. I had gone from a woman who experienced symptoms during exercise to one who popped nitroglycerin like candy because I would have chest pain just walking from one room into another. Even my husband and father—both physicians—couldn't help me. My three boys were terrified that I might die.

I'm sharing this story, not to scare you, but because I am not alone. Unfortunately, there are thousands of women in this country who are misdiagnosed, have delayed diagnosis, or don't receive the appropriate treatment for their heart disease. If you're reading this book, you probably have a story too. And it's important for you to know that you are not alone.

At the time of my diagnosis, I didn't know there was an organization for women like you and me. WomenHeart: The National Coalition for Women with Heart Disease is the only patient advocacy organization serving the eight million American women living with heart disease. It aims to improve the quality of our lives and health care through its support, education, and advocacy. I felt isolated and afraid before I contacted WomenHeart, but the organization referred me to a third cardiologist where I received proper treatment and got my life back. Now I have a normal, busy life. I exercise four to six times a week. I try to rest every day for about ten to twenty minutes, napping, doing crossword puzzles, or reading. And I've found that taking care of myself is not always easy, that I have to work at it on a daily basis.

When you go through an ordeal like this you wonder why. Why is this happening to me? I now know the reason. It happened to me so I could help other women. I vowed that if I ever regained my health, I would become a strong advocate for women and do whatever it took to keep others from enduring what I went through. Now my time is spent as an educator and advocate for other women about heart disease from a grass roots level to a national level.

Little did I know how far my passion would take me. My advocacy work for WomenHeart has taken me to the White House to meet the president and first lady. I have been working with congressional leaders to increase awareness, and put a face on the issue of women and heart disease. Aside from speaking nationally and locally at community and political forums, I have been encouraging medical students and doctors to care for women differently. My story, and the issue of women and heart disease, has been published in national and local newspapers and magazines, such as *Smart Money, Time, The Wall Street Journal, The Washington Post, Biography,* and many others. WomenHeart is a leader in bringing the issue of women and heart disease into the public arena and I am proud to be such an active participant.

For this book, I've interviewed and surveyed more than a hundred women with heart problems from coast to coast, and dozens of health professionals. In quoting these women throughout this book, I haven't used their last names. And unless they requested otherwise, I've changed their first names as well to protect their privacy. My hope is that their stories and advice will help you heal and find answers. If you're a heart patient, I want you to know that I am in this with you and there are millions of other women who share your experience as well. In the weeks and months that follow your heart event, you'll find some days to be easier than other days. And as you might expect, there will be some things in your life that change. This book will help you through the process of change by validating your feelings and by giving you concrete guidance on issues that may arise with heart disease. Through this book, other women heart patients, experts, and I will be there to help you along the way.

Although it may seem like it, heart disease is *not* a death sentence. You can change, grow, and thrive even if you have heart disease. With heart disease, there is hope and there are many things within your control. But it does raise all sorts of questions. Everyone in my life wants the old me back, but I know I will never be the same—how do I let others know I am different? I know exercise and diet are critical to heart health but inwardly I want to rebel against the "shoulds"—how do I fight the inner me? I am still a sexual being but I am scared—how do I get the urge and maintain the interest? My sense of mortality has changed forever—how do I cope with the fear and find hope? How do I feel better about myself? How can I manage my heart disease and have a job/career? And what should I do now, so that I can move on from here? This book is going to answer those questions and many others. It's designed to help you to find the most effective ways possible to cope with the trials and tribulations of heart disease.

This is not a medical book. Women look to their doctors for diagnosis and treatment. I want to provide something that you often don't get at the doctor's office: emotional support. This book is about what I've learned. It's about how to ride the emotional roller coaster that comes with heart disease; how to effectively cope with the kinds of problems that can arise with heart disease; and most importantly how to live well with heart disease. This book is a guide that I needed but couldn't find. My wish is that it will help others to find their way—maybe even you.

PART ONE

BEGINNING THE RECOVERY PROCESS: THE FIRST STEPS

Without a struggle, there can be no progress.

—Frederick Douglass

chapter one

FINDING BALANCE
What Happens When You Go Home

You don't get to choose how you're going to die, or when.
You can only decide how you're going to live now.
—Joan Baez

You're home from the hospital—maybe you're lying in bed or sitting at your kitchen table or taking a shower, and suddenly it hits you, the full weight of what you've been through. And you ask yourself, How do I come to terms with all of this?

Reflecting on your experience, it's as if you're seeing the world in time-lapse photography. You can see yourself going through the chaos of the emergency room—test upon test, one procedure after another, doctors and nurses hovering over you—and then your hospital room with all those tubes and IVs attached to your body. These images seem surreal and disconnected from your real life. You feel like you've been trapped in a scary movie, and you just want to leap off the screen and go home. In the wake of such events, it's not uncommon to experience a sense of shock or feel emotionally numb; these are completely normal reactions to a heart event. And even after you go home, these feelings of shock and numbness may stay with you for a while.

I was terrified when I came home from the hospital. I felt very insecure and fragile. My home didn't feel safe any longer. I felt alone. I was afraid to travel away from home for fear that I would have another cardiac event and my doctor wouldn't be there to "save me." Every now and then I think about the fact that I had a heart attack and will live with the uncertainty of heart disease for the rest of my life. It's all rather overwhelming.

—Joann, Huntington Station, NY, age 59

A heart event isn't just a physical experience. It affects you emotionally too. And once you go home from the hospital you'll begin the task of adjusting to your illness. For most heart patients, this is a time of transition, a time when you're adapting to the new realities you face. Every woman's experience is different. Some women find that their lives will change significantly. Others find that, over time, their daily routines pretty much get back to normal. The degree of change you face will depend on factors such as the severity of your illness, the level of responsibilities you have to take on, and your age and stage of life. But, for just about every heart patient, the process of adapting raises emotional issues. This chapter will touch on those issues. I'm hoping that knowing what's ahead will help you to negotiate these early stages of recovery. I'll also share some advice on how to deal with some of the feelings and experiences you may have, and insights on how to take those first steps towards your emotional and physical recovery.

THINGS ARE DIFFERENT

[My friends and family] tend to remind me not to overtax myself, which gets irritating. I don't like them making a fuss over me. Sometimes I try to listen to them and slow down a little bit. But can't they just let me be?

—Betty, Zanesville, OH, age 58

At some point during or following your hospitalization, you come to know that somehow your life has changed. The realization can feel overwhelming. All of a sudden, you see yourself, your body and your life differently. No matter how you defined yourself before—as a mother, a

homemaker, a businesswoman, a lawyer, a doctor, or a salesperson—
you've transformed. Redefining yourself is an unexpected challenge you
suddenly have to face.

Many women experience a sense of loss. Looking in the mirror, you may
ask yourself: "Who am I now?" The reflection tells you that this experience
has changed your life in ways that are not welcome and not always easy to
process. Whether you're forty-five or sixty-four, before you got sick, you
probably felt like a teenager on the inside. Like most people, you took life
for granted; you felt invincible. That's what most of us believe. It's a healthy,
constructive way to go through life. But now, all of a sudden, you've confronted your own mortality and those internal bubbles filled with images of
yourself have burst. Losing your sense of invincibility disrupts your sense of
security and sense of self, and that can leave you feeling unbalanced. It can
be scary. You tell yourself this is not a club you want to be a member of.
These initial feelings and experiences are normal. Don't worry, over time
you will regain your footing and your hope will be rekindled.

Okay, so that's what's happening inside of you. Then, to make matters
more complex, you're confronted with a flood of mandates from doctors,
health-care providers, and even, at times, from your family and friends:
Take your medications. Go to cardiac rehabilitation. Visit your doctor regularly. Adjust to your physical limitations. Eat right. Exercise. Stop smoking. And find ways to reduce your daily stress. How can anyone reduce
stress, you wonder, when these instructions and changes are making
everything so stressful?

The truth is most heart patients feel overwhelmed at first. As you begin to accept your heart disease, these changes you're being asked to
make won't be as overwhelming as they may seem at first. You'll find
ways to incorporate them into your routine and they'll just become part
of your daily life. Ultimately, you'll accept the new image of yourself as a
heart patient and regain your own internal sense of security. But it's going to take some time and patience. Recognize that change is difficult for
everyone. It's a process of ups and downs. You'd never expect toddlers to
crawl one day, pull themselves up the next, then begin to walk and even
run without difficulty the following day. Well, you can't be expected to
change overnight either. It has to be a gradual process; even adults have
to take courageous baby steps to achieve their goals. You have to take all
these steps one at a time, at your own pace.

There are two ways of meeting difficulties: You alter the difficulties or you alter yourself to meet them.

—Phyllis Bottome, Author

TRY TO SET REALISTIC EXPECTATIONS — OF YOURSELF AND OTHERS

I was depressed because of my inability to care for myself and household in the manner in which I was accustomed. I am a worker, have always been. There was a great stress in my not being able to handle things the way I like them handled.

—Billie, Las Vegas, NV, age 44

It's normal for you and the people who care about you to want things to stay the same—to be the way they've always been. So it's not unusual for your friends and family to set expectations too high. They might hope or even expect that once you're home again, things will go back to normal. And it's not unusual for women heart patients to go home and set the bar too high for themselves. If you set your expectations too high, it can lead to added stress at home and personal disappointment. Everyone's expectations—yours and theirs—can be so unrealistic that you can't possibly meet them.

Here are a few tips to get you through the first weeks at home:

- Go easy on yourself. Don't expect to be able to get right back on track. And don't try to do too much too fast. Studies show that, following a heart attack, women may take on the burden of too many household chores too early in the rehabilitation process. And that can pose a risk of recurrence.[1]
- You'll probably have to change the way things are managed at home and that too will take some time and adjustments. Start small. For example, maybe your partner can get up early once a

---

1. G. L. Rose, J. Suls, P. J. Green, P. Lounsbury, and E. Gordon, "Comparison of Adjustment, Activity, and Tangible Social Support in Men and Women Patients and Their Spouses During the Six Months Post-Myocardial Infarction," *Annals of Behavioral Medicine* 18 (4) (1996): 264–72 FAL.

week to feed the kids, so you can sleep late. Or maybe your kids can take on a daily chore they haven't done before—emptying the dishwasher, taking out the garbage, folding laundry, or even helping with dinner. If everyone pitches in, it will also serve as a daily reminder that you need a little extra support.

- Listen to your body and pay attention. Rest when you need to. Take a nap to rejuvenate during the day. It might be a ten-minute rest or a sixty-minute nap, but do whatever feels right to you. And don't feel guilty about resting.
- Let other people know how you're feeling. If you're tired or feel weak or dizzy, be honest with yourself, your family, and your friends. Don't be afraid to lie down when you need to, even if you have visitors. You need to tell people what your limitations are. You have nothing to gain by overtaxing your body.
- Don't be afraid to ask for help when you need it. Recognize that asking for help is not a sign of weakness. It's a sign of your ability to take control of your life and adapt to new circumstances.
- This is a good time to learn how to say No when you can't do something or need to rest. In fact, setting these limits for yourself and others is an important step toward your full recovery.

RELATING TO YOUR FRIENDS AND FAMILY

Some friends and family are still in disbelief and even denial about my condition. Some have lashed out in anger and rage over my not being the same. I think I was viewed as being very capable. When I appeared ill and became vulnerable, this shook their foundation. I was their glue, the stabilizing force, if you will; then I became unglued.

—Billie, Las Vegas, NV, age 44

Here you are just beginning to deal with your new diagnosis and trying to process the feelings that accompany that experience, and you find relating to your friends and family is at times a struggle. This is a challenge many heart patients face when they go home—how to deal with the other people in their lives; family and friends, the people we all look to for support. To compound the problem, many newly diagnosed patients don't know how to accept support or empathy from others. They have difficulty accepting emotional support because they see it as a sign of weakness or feel that they're being pitied. In fact, people are most likely to tune out empathy from others at those times when they're feeling most vulnerable. In part, it's because those words of comfort and support only serve to confirm the fact that they are sick and they may not be ready for that.

On the flip side of this issue is the ability of friends and family to give appropriate emotional support. Although everyone needs support at times like these, not everyone knows how to be supportive or empathic in a way that may be the most helpful to you. Most people in our lives have good intentions but have never been taught those skills. It's not easy when someone we care about becomes ill and it's also hard to know what to say or what to do to be helpful in that situation. So, sometimes the people who love you the most may fumble a bit in giving support and empathy.

You may not be ready to accept support and empathy; or the people who care about you may have difficulty giving you the support you need. Either way, it can create issues for heart patients—feelings of loneliness and isolation, even distance from the people who care about them the most.

Here's an approach that can help the situation. Recognize that your feelings are pretty raw right now. They probably range from shock and denial to anger and sadness. Most likely your friends and family have not been where you are right now and can only relate to a limited extent to what you are going through. Try gaining some emotional distance from your experience by seeing the situation from the perspective of the people who care about you. Recognize that they're experiencing deep emotions—just as you are. They've been down this frightening path with you; they too wish everything could just be the way it used to be. Their own feelings of helplessness and frustration may be getting in the way of their ability to be supportive, at least supportive in the way you want them to be.

These times are difficult and when your interactions with others break down, the first thing to do is to take a step back and breathe deeply. Take time and think about the fact that you and the people who are close to you are really all in this together. Their experience might be a bit different from yours but it's a loss to them, just as you're experiencing a loss. In all likelihood, your feelings of helplessness and lack of control are what they are experiencing as well. Understanding where they're coming from can help diffuse some of the tension you're feeling and in the long run will make it easier on everyone.

Here's another problem a heart patient encounters. Sometimes, either in response to their out-of-control feelings or in an attempt to be sweet and thoughtful, the people who care about you make comments that make you feel worse instead of better—although that's not their intention. They may think they're showing you that they care by giving you advice, but it doesn't sound that way to you. One of my nurse friends once told me while I was continuing to have chest pain after procedures that my problem could be emotional. She said, "Kathy, I think your heart problems could be in your head instead of your heart—maybe you should get therapy." A few weeks later I ended up with bypass surgery and of course our relationship has never been the same. Other well-meaning comments can also be painful to hear. "Are you sure you should be eating that?" may sound like "Why don't you take better care of yourself? That's how you got into this situation in the first place." Or a statement like "Don't lift that! Please get some rest," implies that you aren't taking proper care of yourself. At times like these, you may think their comments suggest you're the cause of your medical condition—and that your behavior alone will determine whether you get better. What's meant to be supportive and encouraging instead sounds condescending and judgmental, even if their suggestions make sense.

In fact, heart patients know that they're sometimes blamed for their illness and treated quite differently from people with other types of life-threatening diseases. While people with other illnesses are perceived as victims, heart patients may hear comments that suggest they brought it on themselves: "You knew better—why did you smoke?" or, "Gaining weight isn't good for you." For obvious reasons, comments like these aren't terribly helpful and only make you feel worse. Sometimes, the people around you aren't actually coming out and saying such things, but you perceive a lack of empathy or, because you may already feel guilty about your personal habits, you might even imagine they are thinking these things. And these experiences just compound the self-image problems that women face as they age. These feelings can make you feel alone—as if you're not getting the support you need, as if there's no one on your side. Many women heart patients report such feelings.

How should you handle those feelings? First of all, it's important for you to know that the genes you inherited likely played a role in what happened to you. You should not be blamed for your condition. Much of your heart disease was likely beyond your control or you didn't see yourself at risk. But now that you know that you have a heart problem, you will have to work to reduce the risks that you *can* control. Second, it's important to communicate with the people who love you. Your friends and family will need to learn to be patient with you and let you take responsibility for your condition at your own pace. Most newly diagnosed heart patients recognize that they need to change their lifestyles and certain habits. But the people who care about you need to let you grieve about your illness before you can even begin to hear what they have to say.

LEARNING TO COMMUNICATE

So how do you effectively respond to these well-intentioned comments? Ideally, you do so by talking to them, by clearing the air, by clarifying things—clarifying what they're really saying and explaining how it makes you feel. Sometimes heart patients are so emotionally vulnerable from their experience and overwhelmed with feelings that any comment feels like negative criticism. At these times, it is easy to become defensive. Remember that the people who love you are making these comments because they care about you and want you to take care of yourself. They want you to get better. So you need to open up the lines of communication. That means telling them how you feel and hoping they'll be more sensitive. But it also means being aware that you may be emotionally sensitive right now and have a limited perspective.

All that said, a word of caution: Take time to think about the potential consequences of sharing your feelings and thoughts with the person you want to communicate with. Make sure you weigh the pros and cons of having an open discussion with that person. Sometimes no matter how well you communicate your feelings or thoughts, the other person may not accept your openness in the way you had hoped they would. You could be misinterpreted, a conflict could arise or you might not get the kind of response you anticipate.

Remember: Communication is a skill. If you are not a person who communicates your feelings easily, the first time can feel a bit awkward and somewhat scary. To get past the fears, try reminding yourself that communicating with those around you will help you in your healing, recovery, and ultimately with your life. Of course, some people in your life will be easier to talk to than others. You know who they are. They're the good listeners, the ones you feel emotionally close to, the people you can always communicate with. But there will be people who care about you that are not as capable of hearing and understanding your concerns. Those conversations will take more time and patience.

Here's one way to make it easier: Try communicating with "I" messages instead of "you" messages. People tend to respond better if they're not being told that they did something wrong—as in "you're always telling me what to do" or "you're acting like all of this is my fault." Using "I" messages is more constructive and it's much harder for people to argue with them. For example, you might say: "Dad, I know you're concerned about me and I know you're trying to help. But I'm feeling overwhelmed right now. I'm trying to adjust to all the things that the doctor says I need to do. And it makes me feel more overwhelmed when everyone else starts telling me what to do. I just need time to process all of this and figure it out for myself." If you use "I" messages like these, it's more likely that your dad will hear you and not be put on the defensive.

Once you begin the process of communicating, try to learn from it and improve your skills. Ask yourself a few questions. How did your dad respond to your feedback? Did he hear you and acknowledge what you were trying to say? Did he react defensively or did he understand your point of view? From that one conversation, you can learn a lot about your communication style and his listening style.

Even if your first attempts to communicate don't go exactly as you'd hoped, give the communication process time. When it comes to communication, practice really does make perfect. In time, you'll get better at voicing your concerns and the people who care about you should begin to understand how you feel and respond more appropriately. Ultimately, communicating with others will bring you closer to them, so you can work through problems that come between you in the future. Chapter 6 contains more advice on dealing with your family and how to communicate better.

BECOMING PART OF A SUPPORT SYSTEM

The isolation and feelings of being alone are real. I did not think that I could talk to other women who had been through what I had been through. I did not think that I could talk to anyone about my problem. My health-care provider is too busy with other patients to give me the time that I need. Even the cardiologist and specialists are too busy to give their attention. All I get is twenty minutes with the doctor/cardiologist/specialist. That's it. I'm examined like an object and that's it.

—Lila, Juneau, AK, age 58

Your support system can profoundly affect your recovery and reorientation. And often, support seems to elude our grasp. Adjusting to an illness takes time and can be an emotional experience. That's why it's so important to reach out to others who have been where you are right now rather than remain isolated. Reaching out to others is not always easy nor is asserting yourself with those who care about you. But the reality is this: There are millions of women who are experiencing feelings similar to yours. Support groups, group counseling, and connecting to other heart patients via the WomenHeart Internet site can help resolve some of these feelings and give you a way to heal and recover with other women heart patients. And the anonymity of the Web site helps you to feel more comfortable initiating communications with other women. Visiting the WomenHeart Online Community at http://womenheart.clinicahealth.com is one way to hear what other women have to say about their experiences, and for you to share your own.

(See the Resources section for more options.)

TAKING THE FIRST STEPS TOWARD ADDRESSING YOUR RISK FACTORS

Doubtless your doctor has talked to you about your risk factors—those habits and characteristics that put you at risk for heart disease. They range from smoking to being overweight to diabetes. You know your risk factors. In upcoming chapters, I'll talk about long-term strategies for addressing your risk factors, such as diet and exercise. But in the first weeks home, the crucial first steps toward addressing your risk factors involve cardiac rehabilitation and medication management. Those are important first steps you must take to get back on track physically and emotionally.

CARDIAC REHABILITATION IS A MUST

The very first thing that I made the most use of was cardiac rehabilitation. I think it is the best tool to use right away. The education classes, the monitored exercise, talking with other patients, it all helped me to accept my diagnosis and treatment.

—Diana, Des Moines, IA, age 55

One of the most important things you can do for yourself after a heart event is to go to cardiac rehabilitation. The basic goal of cardiac rehabilitation is a permanent change in lifestyle choices—a change that will directly affect your risk factors, whatever they may be. Keep in mind that all of us have risk factors. In fact, according to Dr. Nanette Wenger of Emory University School of Medicine, "The majority of middle-aged and older women in this country have at least one coronary risk factor but they don't know it." There's nothing to feel guilty about, but you may have some work to do to address those risk factors and stay healthy—both physically and emotionally. Cardiac rehabilitation is the first step toward addressing their impact.

Dr. Wayne Sotile, clinical psychologist and author of *Thriving with Heart Disease,* sums up the need for cardiac rehabilitation this way: "Participating in formal cardiac rehabilitation is one of the surest ways to thrive with heart disease." Unfortunately, according to Dr. Sotile, research has shown that women patients are referred less often for this lifesaving intervention than men. Yet because of the unique challenges they face, women stand to benefit from cardiac rehabilitation just as much as, if not more than, men.

Dr. Sotile encourages women to assert themselves with their healthcare providers by calling their offices and getting the necessary referrals to attend cardiac rehabilitation. I asked my cardiac surgeon for a referral to cardiac rehabilitation and he didn't follow through until I contacted his office and made it happen. I can't tell you how many women I have spoken to over the years who have had the same experience. Just think what happens to all of those women who don't assert themselves! The sad fact is that, as a patient, in many cases, if you don't make the effort to make things happen with your own health care then it won't happen.

> *After my heart attack, I did my own research and had to ask my doctor to send me to cardiac rehabilitation. Going through cardiac rehabilitation was my security blanket. I had this fear after the heart attack that any exertion at all and I would drop dead on the spot. Had it not been for the rehabilitation, I believe that I would have gone through a deep depression that so many other women go through. Instead of depression, I came out a fighter, determined to beat the odds and be a role model for other women going through the initial fears of heart disease.*
>
> —Tasha, Hot Springs, AR, age 40

There is no question that there are tremendous psychological, social, and medical benefits for women who attend rehabilitation after their heart event. Readjusting your schedule, getting that referral, and participating in rehabilitation is worth the hassle of getting there.

> *REHAB, REHAB, REHAB!!!! Rehab provides not only exercise, but social interactions, education concerning diet, and more. They also monitor your heart, which provides a sense of comfort and confidence.*
>
> —Judy, Kenai, AK, age 63

Think of cardiac rehabilitation as an investment in you!

MEDICATION MANAGEMENT

> *One of the biggest obstacles I've had to face is accepting the fact that heart medications are necessary to maintain my "quality of life" and not a form of weakness that I need to try to wean myself off of.*
>
> —Ellen, Beverly Hills, MI, age 53

One of the simplest and easiest things you can do for yourself immediately to reduce your risk factors is to take your prescribed medications.

Whatever your doctor has prescribed is designed to help manage your blood pressure, cholesterol, other heart conditions, and/or diabetes. You probably have many different pills that need to be taken at various times of the day. It's really important that you know what each pill is, what it does, the amount of that medicine you're supposed to take and how that physician wants you to take it.

Sadly, over half the people who use medications don't use them correctly. They may be using the wrong over-the-counter medicines or ignoring drug interaction precautions by using one medication that shouldn't be taken with another. Maybe they're taking the right prescription medicine, but they're not following the instructions properly. They're taking too many, or too few, or self-medicating when they decide they need it. Any one of these errors can have serious—or even fatal—consequences. Remarkably, of all hospital admissions, one-tenth of them are due to medication misuse.[2]

That's why it's so important to have direct and open communications not only with your physician but also with your other health-care providers, including your pharmacist. Being your own best health-care advocate is the way to avoid problems. Here are some strategies you can use:

- *Stay informed.* Write down your questions for your doctor or pharmacist before your visits, and then write down their answers, so you don't forget. You want to know: What are the potential side effects? What are potential drug interactions? Should I take this with or without food? Before or after meals? What about alcohol precautions? What do I do if I skip a pill or forget my medication?
- *Avoid mistakes.* Make sure your prescription labels are easy to read and that they state what you're taking the medication for. If not, ask the pharmacist to include this information. Make a list of all the medications you're taking and the dosages, even the ones prescribed by different doctors. Include any vitamins, herbs, and supplements you're taking. Keep this information in an accessible place.

---

2. See www.fda.gov/womens/tttc.htm.

- *Keep your doctor informed.* Be sure to tell your doctor and/or pharmacist about all the medications or supplements you may be taking, including vitamins, minerals, or herbs. Be open and honest about everything you're taking. Let your doctor know about all of your medical conditions or illnesses. And tell your doctor if you're allergic to any medications or have had a problem with any medications that have been prescribed in the past.
- *Don't be afraid to talk about costs.* Let your doctor know if you're concerned about the cost of your medication. Some medications cost less than others. Generic medications may be a less expensive option.
- *Organize your medications.* Buy a plastic pill sorter to help you keep track of your medications. They're inexpensive, available at any drugstore and designed so you can put all of the pills you need for each day in the container. Try to get a size that fits in your purse, so you can keep your pills with you when you're on the go. Your pharmacist can give you advice about the best system for you to use.
- *Use a single pharmacy.* Make sure you go to only one pharmacy for your prescriptions; that will reduce the chance of complications and confusion.
- *Develop a daily routine.* Take your medications at the same time and in same place, if you can. That will help you remember to take pills as prescribed. You'll be less apt to forget to take your pills, which could be dangerous. Like anything else that's new, taking pills is a learned skill—and practice makes perfect. After a while, taking your medications will just become a part of your daily routine. If you forget a pill, call you doctor's office and ask what to do.

What happens if I get side effects from my medications? Should I just stop taking them? The answer is a big No. Stopping your medications abruptly can be harmful if not dangerous to your health. If you are experiencing side effects contact your health-care providers immediately. If they don't get back to you right away, call them as often as necessary to get them to respond to you. Do not delay! It might be a simple matter of adjusting the time of day when you take your medication or you might need to take your medications with food to reduce the chance of nausea. But these are all solutions that need to come from your health-care provider.

For information on clinical trials, online pharmacies, and drug indexes see the Medication Management Resource Guide in the back of this book.

WHAT'S NEXT?

This chapter has given you guidance and support in navigating those first weeks at home and how to take steps towards regaining some of your balance and footing. Now, let's turn our attention back to what's going on inside of you, back to that person looking in the mirror who's asking herself, Who am I now? You may be at the point where you are just realizing it: You've experienced a loss—the loss of your previous perception of yourself. All of these changes and losses are normal and can bring up strong emotions, some akin to grieving, others that are linked to mental health concerns. In the next chapter, I will guide you through how to check your emotional pulse.

chapter two

CHECKING YOUR EMOTIONAL PULSE

What about Your Mental Health?

We need four hugs a day for survival.
We need eight hugs a day for maintenance.
We need twelve hugs a day for growth.
—Virginia Satir, Family Therapist

In this chapter, I'll review some of the stages of grieving, common emotional reactions in the aftermath of a heart event, and symptoms of various mental-health problems that can surface in heart patients. Again, my goal is not to scare you. I want to arm you with the information you need to identify potential problems and seek help before emotional issues become so severe that they interfere with your ability to live well with heart disease. In Chapter 3, I'll provide some guidance on how to go about getting the help you need.

SYMPTOMS THAT ARE COMMON

You've just come home from the hospital and you're noticing changes in your feelings and behavior. Some of these symptoms may include difficulty sleeping, and changes in appetite, mood, and outlook—your feelings about the future. You may also experience irritability, mood swings, a lack of optimism, and feelings of being alone. Don't worry—these reactions are quite common. It's important to recognize that these responses may be linked to grieving, or to your body and mind's way of adjusting to your illness. These are typical reactions and should be short-lived. Short-term coping strategies are discussed elsewhere in this book. They include exercise, stress-reduction techniques, and just plain pampering yourself (see Chapters 4 and 5). I also encourage you to visit the WomenHeart Web site http://womenheart.clinicahealth.com for insights into what other women heart patients have been through and how they've dealt with their reactions.

Problems arise when these common, short-term symptoms go on too long, worsen, and go untreated. If your intense emotions go untreated for too long, you might fall into old habits, such as smoking, overeating, or physical inactivity. And when you have long-term sadness, fear, or anxiety, you may be less likely to follow your doctor's orders regarding medicines, diet, and an overall wellness plan. The bottom line is this: Your emotions are linked to your physical health—and vice versa.

Finding a new sense of self means letting go of some of your old self-perceptions, and that is a process akin to mourning or grieving. Grieving is a natural response to having a heart event. So let me first familiarize you with grieving, so you'll know what to expect. Following that, I'll review some of the common mental-health problems that arise in recovering heart patients.

RECOGNIZING YOUR GRIEF

Even if you've never lost someone you love, you can probably imagine what it feels like. Recovering from such a loss is a painful and arduous process, involving a set of predictable stages. These stages may not always follow one another in exact sequence; they may not all last the same amount of time; and they may not all occur in everyone who experiences grief. But there are certain emotions associated with grief.

Grieving after a heart event is totally normal, even predictable, because you've lost something, for a time at least: your sense of invincibility, your way of living, and your old self. These feelings of grief will probably be most intense in the first year, and the emotions associated with grief—denial, anger, and sadness—will probably come and go. It's important for you to know that these emotions are a perfectly natural response to your situation.

How long will it last? How intense will it be? That depends on a lot of things—your age and phase of life, the extent of the medical trauma you experienced, the physical changes that you endured following your heart event, even your emotional makeup. As you go through the grieving process, you should start to feel better over time. If at some point the suffering feels too intense, or feelings such as sadness or anger are with you all the time, it would be wise to seek counseling. (See Chapter 3 for guidance on how to get help if you need it.)

You'll probably experience some of the different stages outlined in this section of the chapter. I suggest you read through them; that will help you recognize the stage you're going through. The first step is to accept that you're grieving. Allow yourself to let your feelings surface, so you can work through and process them. Then over time you will be able to move on emotionally.

Resisting, pushing down, or avoiding your feelings is like putting a cork stopper in a carbonated drink and then shaking it up. Eventually it will explode. For example, if you feel sad and you don't talk about or acknowledge those feelings, your feelings might surface at unexpected times or in unexpected ways. For example, you might suddenly start to cry uncontrollably in response to a sad news story or during a poignant scene in your child's school play, or even over a minor mishap such as spilling a cup of coffee. Similarly, if you're holding in feelings of anger, you might have an angry outburst that's completely inappropriate—at the office, with a child, or behind the wheel of your car. The point is this: Eventually, those stifled feelings will surface, one way or another.

In addition, ignoring your feelings is not good for your health. People who try to avoid their emotions while grieving are more likely to try to numb themselves with alcohol, drugs, cigarettes, or food, seeking temporary comfort that can ultimately cause more serious health problems. They're also less likely to follow doctor's orders, all of which can add up to greater health risks.

Part of the healing process will begin when you start to forgive yourself. As with many women, you may not have perceived that you had any risk factors for heart disease, and your genes could have played a role as well. You also need to be gentle with yourself and allow time for the emotional healing to take place, no matter how long it takes. Some days you will feel ready to face the world and move on. Other days, you'll just want to bury your head in the sand. There will be times when you'll say: "Forget this. I don't feel like dealing with it. I'm going to do whatever I want." When that happens, try to take a step back. Take time to relax. Take a nap. Read a book. Go to a movie. Treat yourself to a massage or some other indulgence. (See Chapter 5 for more relaxation techniques.) Then try to get back on track. These are times when you should ask your friends and family to give you all the support they can.

Once you get to the other side of your grief, life will be different. But it takes time and patience to get there. At one point or another, you'll probably go through most of the stages described here. Occasionally, you find that you have worked through one stage and then somehow end up there again. Another health problem, a milestone, a seemingly random event, or someone else's illness can trigger a feeling that you're moving backwards emotionally. Holidays, birthdays, the anniversary of your hospitalization, even a visit from an old friend you haven't seen since you've been sick can take you back to a previous stage in the grieving process.

Whatever the cause, revisiting stages is normal. Grief is a fluid, not a stagnant, process. And it will be more intense for some people than others. If you find that you are stuck in one grieving stage for a long period of time, or the intensity of your feelings seems overwhelming, you'll want to seek counseling to work through what is keeping you from moving on.

THE STAGES OF GRIEF

Denial: This can't be happening to me

Denial is generally recognized as the first stage in the grieving process. It's pretty easy to tell if you're in denial. Ask yourself these questions: Do you put off going to the doctor or ignore your symptoms? Do you find yourself not following the doctor's orders? Are other people around you in denial? Do they keep telling you you're fine, when you're not? Are you rebelling against the instructions you've gotten on how to get better? Are you saying to yourself: I don't want to exercise or diet. I just need to take care of business as usual, and get back to my normal routine. If you answered yes to most of these questions, then chances are you are in denial. In Chapter 1, I talked about the feeling that you're in the middle of a scary movie and you just want to jump off the screen, or blink your eyes and go back to your life before this happened. That's denial. And we all go through it.

Denial is a coping mechanism that is our mind's normal defense to help us get through traumatic events. It gives our body and mind a time-out, so we don't have to deal with the full impact of a trauma all at once.

Denial is easy for most women, because many of us have been trained not to talk about our fears, concerns, or worries. So denying the situation comes naturally. In some cases, the people around you may facilitate your denial by sending underlying messages like these: "The worst is over for you." "It looks like you're back on your feet already." "You need to move on." But even if you or the people around you are in denial, at some level you know that eventually you'll have to face the fact that heart disease is part of your life and that some things will have to change.

In truth, denial is a healthy thing—a natural stage in your emotional recovery. It's a way for you to protect yourself. But it can't go on forever. Gradually, at your own pace and when you are emotionally ready, those masked feelings and realities will surface and then you'll proceed to other stages of grief.

Anger: Why is this happening to me?

> There was anger at the years of misdiagnosis. Every time I had to go to the hospital with chest pains there was sadness for my family and for myself. This has been a difficult road. I was told not to work. My identity was taken away. I was young and had no one to talk to about heart disease.
>
> —Rachel, Jamaica, NY, age 52

Once some of the denial subsides, it's not unusual for anger to creep in. Anger is a valuable emotion; if it's expressed in a healthy way, your anger can actually make you feel better. But it can be difficult for women to experience anger, because we've been taught to hold our anger in, that it's unladylike or aggressive or inappropriate, and that we should keep our negative feelings to ourselves. As a result, women tend not to know how to express their anger in a healthy and productive way.

You may not even realize how angry you are until something relatively small catapults you into an angry outburst when you're least expecting it. As I mentioned earlier, when you don't deal with your feelings and instead suppress them, they'll find a way out somehow. You might get angry at your husband or a friend about some little thing, and your reaction perplexes both of you. You might find yourself talking in an uncharacteristically angry tone of voice or having trouble stopping yourself from saying things you regret saying. You might find that you're responding to perceived injustices—some political issue or news items or situation at your child's school—with more gusto and grit than you did before. Or in the worst case scenario, your suppressed anger can surface in the way you discipline your children.

It's important for you to know that anger is a normal part of grieving. But how can you handle it in a healthy way? The best way to deal with it is to express your feelings in words. Try to work through your angry feelings by writing your thoughts down in a journal, or talking to a trusted friend or family member about what's triggering the anger. There may be specific things that happened to you during your heart event that you now realize you're angry about. Maybe a doctor didn't listen to you or someone in your family ignored your illness. Maybe someone treated you carelessly. Sometimes just putting it into words will help you.

Letter writing can be a powerful healing tool to help you manage your anger, particularly if you're angry at a specific person or about a specific incident. You don't necessarily have to send the letter; just writing it will help you release some of your anger. In the introduction, I talked about the Nurse Ratched type who I felt had mistreated me in the intensive care unit (ICU). One of my strategies for dealing with the anger that I felt toward that nurse involved writing a letter to the hospital. The process not only helped me express my anger in a healthy way, but it also inspired the hospital's nursing department to reprimand the nurse and put her in an Employee Assistance Program. The response from the hospital to that one letter validated my experience and my feelings about the nurse's behavior.

Of course, such letters don't always engender such a positive response. If you want to send a letter, be sure to think about the potential consequences, and be ready to face them. You can also have someone else review it, and then get their opinion before you drop it in the mail. But, here's another option that works just as well: Instead of sending the letter, read it out loud and then tear it up, or burn it to symbolically release yourself from the situation that caused you so much pain. You can ask someone close to you to be there while you go through this process. It can be incredibly cathartic—and therapeutic.

Finally and most importantly, you just need to give yourself permission to be angry. You may be angry because of the losses you've experienced: the feeling that your body's let you down, the fact that your life has changed, the sheer fact that you got sick. It's perfectly normal to be asking such questions as, Why did God abandon me and let me down? or Why didn't my doctor catch my heart problems earlier? During the grieving process, anger is really your feelings of helplessness turned inside out.

Just like any other stage of grief, it's possible to get stuck in the anger phase. Recognize that chronic anger is unhealthy physically, socially, and emotionally. So if you find yourself getting angry almost every day for months on end, you'll want to seek help from a doctor or mental-health specialist to get yourself back on track.

Guilt: Did I bring this on myself? Did I make my family suffer?

> I "dropped out" as a mother and a wife [following my heart event]. My husband filled in. Finding my way back to motherhood took me the longest because I was so self-absorbed in my illness. I certainly did become a dedicated wife and mother eventually and we did talk about this in therapy, too. My guilt is I think my youngest son missed out on a lot of mothering during an important time in his childhood. He'll probably be in therapy someday to overcome the repercussions.
>
> —Irene, Springfield, NJ, age 51

Heart patients inevitably feel guilty about having heart disease. And they also have guilt about their family and friends, who might have been affected by their emotional storm. They feel responsible for their condition, whether they could have prevented it or not. Feelings of guilt are also a natural part of the grieving process.

The first step in alleviating guilt is to start forgiving yourself. That's not always as easy as it sounds. You need to be patient and gentle with yourself, and recognize that you are only human. It may be helpful at this stage to remind yourself, again, that you didn't know that you had risk factors for heart disease, that most women your age have risk factors, and that circumstances beyond your control—including your genetic predisposition—played a role in your illness. Even women who knew they had risk factors before their heart event need to forgive themselves. Try to look at it this way: You've been given a second chance to live a healthier lifestyle. And remember, everyone has habits that can contribute to heart disease. At this point, it will be helpful to begin to address those habits. When you start to change the behavior that you feel guilty about, the guilt will begin to subside.

Start small. Make a list of all of the things you want to change about yourself that may have contributed to your heart event. Pick a few key items on your list, and then set realistic, small, and incremental goals. For instance, if your goal is to change your eating habits, your list might include buying leaner meats, using olive oil instead of butter, cutting down on your sweets, and eliminating fatty foods. At this point, it would be helpful to consult with a dietician or nutritionist for advice. If your doctor doesn't refer you to one, be assertive and ask for a referral. Your dietician can help you to slowly negotiate those important stages of change and set realistic and achievable goals. There's more about diet strategies in Chapter 4, but for now the idea is this: To begin alleviating your guilt, you've got to take the first small steps toward changing your habits. If your goal is to stop smoking, begin by looking into all the ways you can approach quitting. Make a list of what you can do and then take the first steps toward doing it, whether that means joining a smoking-cessation program or trying nicotine gum or talking to your doctor about ways to quit.

No matter what habit you choose to address, the first step is always the hardest. But once you actively do something, your guilt will begin to subside. Of course, change takes time and you'll have many days where you'll move in a positive direction and then other days when you'll think you are going backwards. This is normal. If you have a setback, be gentle with yourself—and forgiving.

You may find that you have other sources of guilt. Sometimes mothers feel guilt related to their children. They may be afraid that they've passed heart disease on to their kids or they may experience guilt related to a grown child who has to make some lifestyle changes to take care of them. You may feel guilty that you can't carry on your household responsibilities or carry the same load professionally. And, of course, if you have a husband or partner, there may be some feelings of guilt that center on that relationship. All these issues are addressed extensively in Chapter 6.

The most important thing to remember is to go easy on yourself. The positive side of feeling guilty is that it can inspire you to change unhealthy habits and behaviors. And by getting past it, you move on to the next stages of grieving.

Fear and Bargaining: Please don't let me die. I promise I'll do better from now on

We all know what bargaining is, because we've all done it at some point during our illness. Bargaining usually happens during your most intense moments of fear and anxiety. (I promise, God, if you make me healthy, I'll do anything you want.) We bargain with our doctors. (I'll come in for another stress test today, but if I have to be catheterized, can I go home and talk to my kids first?) We bargain with our families and with our children. (I'll take you to your friend's house later, if you'll just let me take a nap right now.) Bargaining is a way of trying to gain control in a seemingly uncontrollable situation. It's a way of dealing with your fears. And fear is another natural response to what we, as heart patients, experience.

During the first year of your recovery, once you get past denial, fear can rear its ugly head. It's a perfectly natural and healthy response; it means you're facing your illness head-on and confronting your fears about the future. You worry: What if I have another heart attack? What if I get worse? Or maybe even: What if I die? Talk about it—to a friend or family member, a pastor or rabbi, a grief counselor or therapist. Talking about your fears can make those feelings more manageable and less scary.

> *Don't fight yourself, talk to someone. Get any questions you have answered by the appropriate person for that question. I found someone to talk to about dying. Just getting those issues out in the open is so helpful. It is okay to be afraid but not okay to stay afraid.*
> —Diana, Des Moines, IA, age 55

Knowing that fear is part of the grieving process gives you permission to work through and talk about it. Recognize that these are normal feelings and that addressing them will help you move forward in your recovery.

After my heart attack I had no idea how I would go back to being a mom, wife, and loan officer at the bank. I was afraid to go from one floor of my house to another without nitroglycerin in my pocket. Going from home to my office in New York terrified me. I was sure I would drop dead on the street and no one would help me. The fears were endless.

—Irene, Springfield, NJ, age 51

Fear is a natural reaction. But if your fears become so intense that they are debilitating or if you get stuck in this stage of the grieving process, you should seek counseling. Irene describes her fears as "endless." The depth of those fears led her to seek help. Irene found that just by talking through her fears with a therapist, she was able to get past them and move to the next stage of grief.

Another valuable way of dealing with your fears involves gathering all the information you can about whatever it is that's frightening you. Say your doctor wants to do an angioplasty, and you don't really know what that means. That can be scary. Some patients find it reassuring to read about the procedure. But whatever you do, don't just go online and Google "angioplasty" or randomly search for information. That can get even scarier, because there's no guarantee that the information you find will be accurate. Instead, ask your doctor to recommend some resources—books, articles, and Web sites—or visit a site like WomenHeart that you know is reliable. (See Chapter 9 for more details on getting your medical questions answered.)

Just remember that you can't escape your feelings. Confronting your fears by talking about them or arming yourself with information can help alleviate anxiety, and that's important for your physical well-being. Empower yourself by communicating and by dealing directly with your fears.

Sadness: I'm not the same person anymore

As you move through the stages of grief, you begin to adapt to a new reality. When you reach the stage where you consciously accept the fact that you have heart disease, that you will be a heart patient for the rest of your life, and that you are a different person, you may experience sadness. The sadness comes from knowing that you have lost your old images of yourself and now have to formulate some new images. This stage is central to the grieving process. Although that knowledge in itself probably doesn't make you feel any better, it may be helpful to know that sadness means you are beginning to emerge from your grief and that you are turning an important corner.

This is where you begin to give yourself permission to be a different person. You can begin to recognize that things have changed for you physically and emotionally—and that's the true first step toward acceptance. You are doing the difficult emotional work that's necessary to get you where you need to be. You're making progress toward accepting the new you.

> *You must grieve the loss of the "old" you. I just think you have to acknowledge it and learn as many coping skills as you can. I don't like it when I am a bit down, but I also understand this mood will soon pass. I just try to do my favorite things during this down time.*
>
> —Ashley, Phoenix, AZ, age 48

How do you cope with the sadness, the internal turmoil, and moodiness that come with losing your sense of self? First of all, it's important to face and experience your sadness. It can be valuable to just lie down and let the sadness seep over you; don't try to escape or ignore the feelings. This may well be the deepest stage of grieving, because you are truly mourning what you have lost. Talking with someone can help, just as it helped you work through some of the other stages of grief. Remember, typically, the most intense period of grieving lasts no more than a year—meaning that, although you may revisit some of these stages again, you will probably pass through most of them and complete the grieving cycle in the first twelve months following your diagnosis. So this sadness you're experiencing will go away and, even during the most intense phase, it won't be with you every moment of every day. On the other hand, if you find you have prolonged and unrelenting sadness that is with you all the time and doesn't ever seem to go away, be sure to see a counselor or mental-health professional. Later in this chapter you will get the guidance you need on how to distinguish between the natural sadness that is part of your recovery process and bona fide depression.

Mobilization, Hope, and Acceptance: I am ready to move on

Working through all these stages takes energy, time, and patience. Mobilizing yourself, having hope, and accepting your illness is the next stage, and it is empowering. You begin to think of yourself as a survivor, and begin to wear your heart disease as a badge of courage and honor. You no longer feel beaten by your disease, but think of yourself as a woman who can make your own life better. At this point, some women begin to consider helping other heart patients.

> *The turning point has finally happened, even though my heart disease is not getting better. I have hope because of the women that I have met and the work I can do for WomenHeart. Running the support group and going out on speaking engagements has finally gotten me to the point of acceptance. Would I choose this illness? No, but there are a lot worse things that could have happened to me. The friendships I have formed are from having heart disease. I would not have met such caring, loving women otherwise. I am stronger today than I have ever been in my life. I feel empowered.*
>
> —Rachel, Jamaica, NY, age 52

This is the stage of grieving when women are able to face their illness head-on, embrace their limitations, and fortify their strengths. This is the light at the end of the tunnel, the stage when you'll feel as if you're coming out of a horrific storm and finding a bright, warm, sunny path ahead.

Everyone's experience is different, but this is the point in your emotional journey where you begin to feel as if you have a new life. Women report a sense of peace, hopefulness, and relief. You've been through these difficult emotional and physical stages of your illness, and you're ready to accept the new person that you've become. You become less self-concerned and more comfortable reaching out to others.

> *I think it is better not to focus solely on yourself [while taking care to improve your health]. Taking care of one's family, working at something you enjoy, having good friends, and most of all a loving family truly helps. I find that even though new health is-*

sues aside from heart disease arise, as I grow older, I'm not afraid.
I have faith that somehow I'll be able to survive.

—Nancy, New York, NY, age 74

Now that I have familiarized you with the stages of grieving, what do you do if you think your emotional state is linked to something more serious?

WHEN IT'S MORE THAN GRIEF

Women need to know that they are at risk for depression and other psychological problems after developing an acute illness that then becomes a chronic illness. Living with a chronic illness can affect emotional states. Unfortunately, research shows that psychological reactions to illness are not cared for as well as blood pressure and cholesterol. All women need to be able to identify the signs of stress, anxiety, sadness, depression, and talk to their health-care providers for referrals to counseling and other support programs.

—Kathy Berra, MSN, Clinical Trial Director at the Stanford Prevention Research Center

You can't expect to feel quite like yourself in the weeks and months following a heart event. After all, your body's been through a lot—and you've been through a lot. In fact, it's not at all uncommon for women heart patients to have intense emotional responses to their experiences. In one study, more than half of women heart patients reported having some kind of mental health issue due to their experiences with heart disease.[1] Heart patients may have depression, anxiety, and other mental-health problems that can range from mild to severe.

A woman's genes, family and social supports, her lifetime experiences and personal history, even the developmental stage she is in when her heart trouble surfaces will all influence her emotional response. If you

---

1. E. Marcuccio, N. Loving, S. K. Bennett, and S. N. Hayes, "A Survey of Attitudes and Experiences of Women with Heart Disease," *Women's Health Issues* 13 (2003): 23–31.

have a history of anxiety, depression, or other psychological difficulties, coping with the aftershock of a heart event may be particularly difficult. You know yourself better than anyone—and you know the symptoms. Be sure to consult your mental-health professional at the first sign of a problem. And for those of you with no history of psychological problems, if you think these mental-health issues are affecting you, seeking treatment is critical for your overall recovery. First, remind yourself that you are not alone—mental-health issues can be a natural consequence of your experiences with heart disease. Second, even if you are unsure about what is happening to you emotionally, it is better to be evaluated by a mental-health professional than to suffer in silence. But all too often women ignore their emotional symptoms when they arise and fail to seek help when they need it. You and your doctor may be so focused on your physical health that emerging mental-health issues don't even get noticed. You may have to be your own best advocate and ask for the help you need.

Recognize that your physical health is linked to your mental health. It's important to keep in mind that if you're sixty years old or younger you are at a greater risk of becoming depressed after a heart attack than older women or men in any age group.[2] There seems to be a biological interaction between heart disease and mental-health problems such as depression and anxiety. The biological and hormonal changes that occur with depression seem to be correlated with increasing heart problems.[3] It's important to keep this interaction in mind and recognize that you may not be able to completely control your mental-health responses to your heart disease by sheer force of will.

If your emotions overwhelm you, they can interfere with your ability to take care of yourself. The more closely you follow your doctor's orders, the more likely it is that your physical health will improve. And a mental-health issue can get in the way of that process, making it harder to stick with essential lifestyle changes related to eating, exercise, smoking, or other health-related habits. In short, there is help available and it's effective—by reaching out to friends, family, and clergy, or getting counseling,

2. Susmita Mallik, et al., "Depressive Symptoms After Acute Myocardial Infarction: Evidence for Highest Rates in Younger Women," *Archives of Internal Medicine* 166 (2006): 876–83.

3. D. E. Kemp, M. Shishuka, K. N. Franco, et al., "Heart Disease and Depression: Don't Ignore the Relationship," *Cleveland Clinic Journal of Medicine* 70 (9) (2003): 745–61.

therapy, or psychiatric treatment. In getting that support you need, you will be helping yourself to heal. (See Chapter 3 regarding how to find help when you need it.)

Major depression is one of those mental-health challenges that some heart patients encounter. It is important to know about depression, so if necessary, you can take steps do something about it.

DEPRESSION AND HEART DISEASE

Research has demonstrated a very real connection between heart disease and depression. In fact, studies show that one in three people develop major depression following a heart attack.[4][5] People who have heart disease are more likely to experience depression and, conversely, people who are depressed have a greater chance of developing heart disease.[6] How common is depression among women with heart disease? Studies suggest that depression occurs in 18 to 20 percent of people with heart disease who have not had a heart attack; and it occurs in 40 to 65 percent of people who have experienced a heart attack.[7] Add to that the fact that, in the general population, women are twice as likely as men to develop depression[8] and the answer is clear: Very common. Given that there are eight million women with heart disease, you can begin to imagine the number of women heart patients who develop depression.

It is very important to seek medical help if you are experiencing depression. Research shows that even heart attack survivors who have

4. D. A. Reiger, W. E. Narrow, D. S. Rae, et al., "The De Facto Mental and Addictive Disorders Service System. Epidemiologic Catchment Area Prospective 1-Year Prevalence Rates of Disorders and Services," *Archives of General Psychiatry* 50 (2) (1993): 85–94.

5. F. Lesperance, N. Frasure-Smith, and M. Talajic, "Major Depression Before and After Myocardial Infarction: Its Nature and Consequences," *Psychosomatic Medicine* 58 (2) (1996): 99–110.

6. C. B. Nemeroff and D. L. Musselman, "Depression and Cardiac Disease," *Depression and Anxiety* 8, suppl. no. 1 (1998): 71–79.

7. National Mental Health Association, "Co-Occurrence of Depression with Medical, Psychiatric, and Substance Abuse Disorders," http://www.nmha.org/infoctr/factsheets/28.cfm (accessed June 2005).

8. National Mental Health Association, "Depression in Women," MHIC Factsheet: Depression-Depression in Women, http://www.nmha.org/infoctr/factsheets/23.cfm (accessed June 2005).

THE SIGNS OF CLINICAL DEPRESSION

If you have at least five of these symptoms, nearly every day for at least two weeks, or others notice these changes, you should seek help:

- Persistent feelings of being sad or empty.
- Diminished interest and pleasure in all or most normal daily activities.
- Significant weight gain or loss due to changes in appetite.
- Changing sleep habits—either an increase or decrease.
- Feelings of restlessness, agitation, or being slowed down.
- Fatigue or loss of energy.
- Feelings of inappropriate or excessive guilt and worthlessness.
- Difficulty thinking, making decisions, or concentrating.
- Recurring thoughts of death or suicide.

Source: National Institutes of Mental Health and Diagnostic and Statistical Manual of Mental Disorders—Fourth Edition

minimal depressive symptoms are more likely to die after a heart attack than those who are not depressed.[9] In much the same way that stress affects your body, depression can result in increased blood pressure; it can affect your heart rhythms; it can increase stress hormones and affect clotting, which can lead to a heart attack.[10] [11] In addition, those of us who experience a major depression are less likely to take good care of ourselves and take the steps that are necessary to get better. A depressed person may lack the discipline to take essential medications, go to cardiac rehabilitation, and adopt heart-healthy habits. That can lead to medical setbacks. If depression goes untreated, it can spin out of control, leading to suicidal feelings.

If you are thinking or talking about suicide, the most important thing to do is to tell someone. Go directly to the emergency room and get help. No matter how you feel now, those feelings will change over time—once

---

9. Kemp et al., "Heart Disease."

10. Ibid.

11. National Institute of Mental Health, "Depression and Heart Disease," NIH Publication No. 02–5004 (posted June 17, 2002).

you get help. That's the thing about mental-health troubles. Initially they might seem insurmountable. But in reality most mental-health problems are treatable and curable.

Remember, mental-health issues are *health* issues. Depression is a medical condition. And it is treatable. The vast majority of those who receive treatment with medication, psychotherapy, or combinations of both get better.[12] The key is to get treatment as soon as possible. (See Chapter 3, Getting the Help You Need.)

Unfortunately depression can be hard to identify—in those you love and in yourself.

> *At one point my friend, Jean, said that I reminded her of her husband. He had lost his sense of humor for nearly a year after a very serious cancer operation and long recovery. I had always been an optimistic, idealistic kind of person. And when Jean said that, I realized my newfound cynicism, like his humorlessness, was a symptom of depression. They were just different manifestations of the same illness. Jean's husband got back his sense of humor and I eventually returned to my former idealism. But it took nearly a year.*
>
> —Lucy, New York, NY, age 59

Try to stay alert to the symptoms of depression following a heart event. Talk to your health-care provider about how you feel emotionally as well as physically. Unfortunately, sometimes depression goes undiagnosed and untreated in heart patients, because symptoms such as sleeping difficulties and change in appetite may look like normal responses to your heart event.[13]

It may be difficult for you, your family, your friends, and even your doctors to tweeze out the warning signs of depression. Check for the symptoms listed on page 34. If you suspect you have depression, it's better to err on the side of caution. Don't hesitate to see your doctor.

---

12. National Institute of Mental Health, D/ART Campaign, "Depression: What Every Woman Should Know," NIH Publication No. 00–4779, 2000.

13. National Mental Health Association, "Co-Occurrence of Depression with Medical, Psychiatric, and Substance Abuse Disorders," http://www.nmha.org/infoctr/factsheets/28.cfm (accessed June 2005).

ANXIETY DISORDERS

*I was afraid to be alone or where I couldn't get help. When I was
at home alone, I would leave my front door unlocked just in case I
needed emergency help. I was also afraid to drive alone. Two of my
events had happened when I was driving.*

—Marilyn, Palm Desert, CA, age 62

Many recovering heart patients experience anxious or depressive moods
or anxiety disorders. That's understandable. Your sense of well-being has
been shaken. Even if you don't have major depression, as a recovering heart
patient you are vulnerable to a variety of anxiety disorders that may be related to the impact of the disease. In fact, 40 to 65 percent of heart attack
survivors, over time, experience intermittent anxious or depressive moods.[14]

But how do you tell the difference between mild anxiety and fear and
having a full-blown anxiety disorder? How do you distinguish between
worrying—something we all experience—and an anxiety disorder, a condition requiring treatment? It's not easy to diagnose yourself. Anxiety disorders involve excessive, constant worrying that interferes with your daily
activities; it may be so intense that you're paralyzed with fear. The symptoms worsen progressively over time; they may come out of the blue; and
they have no real identifiable cause. Anxiety disorders interfere with the
quality of our day-to-day lives. It's not unusual for women who experience anxiety disorders to be depressed as well,[15] all of which can stop us in
our tracks.

There's no reason to suffer needlessly or try to tough it out. If you can't
shake your feelings of fear and anxiety, the best solution is to see a mental-
health professional. Anxiety is the most common mental-health disorder
in America.[16] Anxiety disorders have a variety of names and symptoms.

---

14. Kemp et al., "Heart Disease." S. J. Schleifer, M. M. Macari-Hinson, D. S. Coyle,
et al., "The Nature and Course of Depression Following Myocardial Infarction,"
Archives of Internal Medicine 149 (1989): 1785–89.

15. D. A. Regier, D. S. Rae, W. E. Narrow, et al., "Prevalence of Anxiety Disorders
and Their Comorbidity with Mood and Addictive Disorders," *British Journal of
Psychiatry Supplement* 34 (1998): 24–28.

16. National Mental Health Association, "Anxiety Disorders," Anxiety Disorders-
Anxiety Disorders (General), http://www1.nmha.org/camh/anxiety/
anxdis.cfm (accessed January 2007).

They have one thing in common: They all respond well to treatment with medication, psychotherapy, or a combination of both. With appropriate care, 90 percent of people recover from anxiety disorders.[17]

In the Introduction, I described my experiences leading up to a diagnosis of post-traumatic stress disorder (PTSD), which is an anxiety disorder. Following a heart attack, some women experience PTSD, which can include such symptoms as recurring memories or nightmares about the heart attack; emotional distress when they pass by hospitals or on the anniversary of the heart attack; and becoming distant and detached. PTSD is just one example of severe anxiety sparked by a heart-related event.

Regardless of whether your feelings of anxiety are mild or severe, you owe it to yourself to look into it. Avoid evaluating yourself. Let an expert do that. See a doctor, psychotherapist, or psychiatrist for an evaluation. You won't be sorry. Recognizing a possible mental-health condition and doing something about it is the first step to recovery—and a sign of our ability to manage all the other changes that we have to make in our lives to thrive as heart patients.

TAKING ACTION

This chapter has familiarized you with the stages of grieving and other mental-health concerns that commonly affect heart patients. No matter where you are on the emotional spectrum, getting help from a mental-health professional can have a tremendous positive impact. Chapter 3 will give you guidance on how and when to get the help you need. It includes step-by-step instructions on how to choose the right treatment and select a therapist that fits your needs—including guidance on how to interview a mental-health professional.

17. Anxiety Disorders Association of America, "Brief Overview of Anxiety Disorders," http://www.adaa.org/GettingHelp/BriefOverview.asp (accessed April 28, 2005).

chapter 3

GETTING THE HELP YOU NEED

*One of the most valuable things we can do to heal
one another is listen to each other's stories.*
—Rebecca Falls, Author

FACING THE SOCIAL STIGMA

The first step to getting professional help for mental-health concerns is abolishing the stigma that goes with it. Heart disease also has a stigma, which compounds the problem and makes it difficult for women heart patients to think positively and willingly accept help. Self-sabotage is not uncommon: "I've got heart disease because of my lifestyle choices. Now I think I'm losing it and have to go for help, when I've created the problems in the first place. So why should I get help? I'm too far gone." Or "I don't know where to start." Or even: "It's my own fault."

So how do you get beyond this type of thinking? Many women have been socialized not to ask for or accept help. Some women have been taught that getting help is a sign of weakness. Others think that if they get therapy that means they are going crazy. According to a study conducted by the National Mental Health Association, more than half the women surveyed claimed that *denial* kept them from getting treatment for mental-health issues; 41 percent of the women reported that *embarrassment* or *shame* kept them from seeking help.[1] A woman heart patient can only live well with heart disease and seek out the treatment she needs when she no longer embraces those negative thoughts. And those thoughts have a profound effect on women who seek treatment. One study showed *that only half of the women who experience clinical depression ever seek treatment.*[2] Similarly, *only one-third of the women with anxiety disorders seek treatment.*[3]

Women are notorious for taking care of everyone else in their lives and, all too often, they put their own needs last. A study conducted by Procter & Gamble in 2000 showed that, in the hierarchy of women's concerns, women put their children, home, careers, pets, and spouses ahead of themselves and their own health—in that order.[4] It makes an enormous difference in women's lives when they change their priorities and put their health-care needs closer to the top of the list—and that includes mental health-care needs.

Becoming a heart patient is a wake-up call. Women have to find the strength within to identify their needs, and to ask and demand that those needs be met. Think of yourself as the glue that holds your family together. What happens if you can't function normally and the glue disintegrates? If you were a wounded survivor of a battle, you'd have those wounds treated, wouldn't you? Your psyche is no different and needs to heal too, just like your body. Getting treatment for mental-health concerns should not be viewed as any different from getting medical help for a physical illness. It's important to recognize that mental-health treatment is central to the overall recovery process.

MAINTAINING PRIVACY

As a psychotherapist, I've found that many of my clients were concerned that their friends and family would judge them for getting mental-health

---

1. National Mental Health Association, "Depression in Women," http://www.nmha.org/infoctr/factsheets/23.cfm (accessed June 2005)

2. Ibid.

3. Anxiety Disorders Association of America, "Brief Overview."

4. Mayo Clinic/Hierarchy of Female Concerns. P&G 2000 Health Archetype Study.

treatment. Attitudes about therapy and medication vary dramatically from one person to another—depending on regional and cultural attitudes, or simple differences in how people have been raised. Based on television and the movies, you might think that everyone in urban America has a therapist. On the other hand, experience tells me that therapy is not so widely accepted everywhere. Depending on your attitudes, and those of your friends and family, you might be worried about what people will think.

The wonderful thing about mental-health treatment is you have the absolute right not to tell a soul that you're getting help. Your privacy is yours to protect. You can be as selective as you want to be about with whom you share your personal information. So if you don't want people to know you're seeing a therapist or psychiatrist, you can choose to keep it confidential. Treat the subject as you would treat any private information. Share it only with people you wish to share it with, people you feel you can trust. That's your decision to make.

As a general rule, if you feel the least bit uncomfortable sharing personal information with a friend or family member, that's probably a sign that you shouldn't share it. Trust your instincts. Privacy is a legitimate concern and if you're conflicted or feel guilty about not revealing your personal information to a friend or relative, you should feel free to discuss it with your therapist. He or she can help you deal with these issues.

The important thing to remember is not to let your attitudes or your family's attitudes about therapy get in the way of seeking treatment when you need it. According to the National Mental Health Association, at any given moment, 54 million Americans have a mental-health issue of some type that requires treatment.[5] Yet only eight million actually seek the help they need. There may be a million individual reasons that people don't address their mental-health issues. But I'd be willing to bet that attitudes are one of them.

As heart patients, we don't have the luxury of letting attitudes get in our way. We owe it to ourselves to take care of our mental health so it doesn't impede our recovery. Once we get past the social stigma, we're on our way. We can begin to get the help we need and greatly improve our chances of living well with heart disease.

---

5. National Mental Health Association Fact Sheet, "Mental Health Statistics," http://www.nmha.org/infoctr/factsheets/15.cfm (accessed September 2006).

Just Do It

Your doctor has probably recommended exercise as part of your recovery program. The good news is that exercise has numerous benefits. Exercise can decrease stress. It can help you sleep better at night. And it increases the sense that you have control over your life. Studies also suggest that exercise might actually reduce depressive symptoms and improve mood.[6] So there's one thing you can do immediately to improve your attitude: Follow the exercise regimen recommended by your doctor. It should improve your mental health as well as your heart health.

Actively Challenge Yourself Every Day

No matter how you're feeling it's important to do a few things every day to keep yourself moving and functioning. Get out of bed every day and challenge yourself with small, achievable goals and responsibilities. You might start by just doing more and more of your normal, daily activities every day. Just the process of moving and doing—and not thinking too much about it—will enhance your mood. If you think too much, these tasks might take on a life of their own and seem insurmountable. If you don't fight the urge to do nothing, then you set yourself up for a self-fulfilling negative thinking and reinforce feelings of helplessness.

Here's a constructive approach for stopping negative thinking in its tracks.

- If you find it difficult to get out of bed, set a time limit on your rest periods and periods of intense emotions; then just get up and try to move forward again.
- Try writing in a journal to express your unfiltered feelings and then reading what you've written out loud. It can be remarkably therapeutic to listen to your feelings spoken. It will give you a different perspective.

---

6. C. B. Taylor, J. Sallis, and R. Needle, "The Relationship Between Physical Activity and Exercise and Mental Health," *Public Health Report* 100 (1985): 195–201.

- Use that information to plan a course of action about how to improve your outlook. Start small. Such plans might include going out to lunch with some friends, going to speak to your favorite clergy, taking a walk, going out and digging in your garden, or doing something you've always wanted to do but never made the time.

- Write your plans down and decide how to implement them to improve your mood. These should be small, realistic, and achievable goals.

- Then act on your ideas by taking one step at a time. For instance, one idea might be to take an adult education course at a community center or local college. First you'll want to explore what's available. Then you'll want to see how it meshes with your schedule and finances. Then, once you've reviewed the options, you can sign up for a course. Finally, you'll begin taking the course.

- Every step forward in the process should invigorate you and improve your mood. Just as importantly, as you bring your plans to life, they'll not only affect your daily routine, they'll also have a positive impact on you.

TAKE THE NEXT STEP

I immediately knew that I was depressed and I had never had a depressed day in my life prior to heart surgery. I went to a male psychologist and then a male psychiatrist and received no help. They noted my symptoms, prescribed medication, but never discussed my heart disease with me. I thought I was going to die; we planned for my death; we sold our home and moved into a condo. It was a terrible experience. Then I went to a female psychiatrist. She listened and discussed my feelings with me. Eventually, she prescribed medication and after six weeks, I was feeling like myself again. This process took one and a half years—getting treated properly for the depression. Today because of antidepressants and counseling I feel great!

—Linda, Maitland, FL, age 59

In Chapter 2, I reviewed the symptoms of depression, anxiety, and other mental-health problems that can come in the wake of a heart event. If you're concerned about your mental health, there are two things to keep in mind. First, it's dangerous for you to try to diagnose and/or treat yourself. Second, if you think you might need help, there's no harm in exploring the possibility of getting treatment. What do you have to lose? In suffering, all we do is encumber our ability to reach our potential. Life is too short for that.

The first step is simple: See your medical doctor for an evaluation. Your physician can help determine whether or not your symptoms are linked to a health problem, a mental-health problem, some combination—or even a hormonal issue. Perimenopausal and menopausal women may be experiencing depression, anxiety, or mood swings that are related to the hormonal changes their bodies are going through, which may require an entirely different approach to treatment. Regardless of the root cause, you owe it to yourself to see a doctor.

> *I learned that much of what I was feeling was pretty common among women and clearly contained elements of depression. It is difficult to figure out what is causing the symptoms. I am at that wonderful perimenopausal age and trying to figure out if things are hormone related, heart related, or something else entirely. It is pretty confusing.*
>
> —Ellen, Beverly Hills, MI, age 53

Your health-care provider is best qualified to accurately assess what's going on and diagnose the problem. Then you can address it together. If it is a mental-health issue, you and your doctor can determine what type of treatment is best for you—medication, some form of therapy, or a combination of both. That will depend, in part, on the severity or type of depression or anxiety you are experiencing. The more severe the depression or anxiety, the more likely your doctor will recommend medication. Medications can help modify your symptoms. Psychotherapy is helpful for mild to moderate depression and certain anxiety disorders. And therapy will help you to learn more effective coping techniques to manage your troubles. For some of us, a combination of medication and psychotherapy may be the best approach.

Keep in mind: When there's more than one mental-health provider involved, it's critical that there be a team approach. From the very beginning, close communication between you and all the providers involved—including your medical doctor—will lead to a more effective treatment, and ensure that there are no drug interaction issues involving your heart medications and any psychotherapeutic medications that you are taking.

THERAPY

> *I was aware of my depression and am being treated through therapy and no medication. I probably should be medicated but I take fourteen pills and four shots a day . . . I think I'm at my limit for medications right now. Besides, I like the therapy—it gives me the chance to talk about it and I don't get to do that anywhere else—not even at home.*
>
> —Sarah, West Hempstead, NY, age 29

Again, before seeking psychotherapy, see your physician for an evaluation—so he or she can help determine whether your symptoms are linked to a health problem, a mental-health problem, or both. There are many different types of mental-health problems in which depression and/or anxiety can be a component. That's one reason why it's so important to seek professional help as soon as possible—so you can get an accurate diagnosis and effective treatment.

If psychotherapy is recommended, you may be referred to one of the following for treatment: a psychiatrist, psychologist, clinical social worker, licensed professional counselor, certified drug and alcohol counselor, nurse psychotherapist, marital and family counselor, or counselor affiliated with the clergy. There are many types of therapists and therapies with just as many theoretical approaches, treatment styles, and time frames for treatment.

FINDING A THERAPIST

Only you can choose a therapy that is right for your recovery. Given that, interviewing a potential therapist is not only appropriate, it's essential. Learn as much as you can. Try to familiarize yourself with the different

TYPES OF THERAPY

Cognitive-behavioral therapy focuses on changing our thinking and our patterns of behavior. This is a short-term, time-limited therapy. It may include biofeedback, stress management, and relaxation techniques. Homework may be assigned. Generally, the therapist sets goals, and develops plans and treatment strategies with the patient. This type of therapy is shown to be effective in treating both anxiety disorders and depression.

Psychodynamic psychotherapy (also known as *insight-oriented therapy*) has its roots in Freudian theories. This is a long-term therapy that involves bringing the unconscious into consciousness to provide insight and resolve internal conflicts. There may not seem to be a lot of direct one-to-one responses to your concerns by the therapist. The process and the relationship between the therapist and the client are central to the therapy.

Humanistic therapy is rooted in Rogerian, Gestalt, and existential theories. This is a client-centered therapy, so the focus is on respecting and enhancing each client's unique and individual qualities. The goals are to help each client reach their potential through self-directed change and growth. The therapist mirrors the client and helps the client to see his or her own answers.

Eclectic therapy simply means the therapist uses multiple theories and techniques. Eclectic therapists tend to be very actively engaged. It is a multifaceted approach and may be based on your unique needs and concerns.

Interpersonal therapy is a short-term therapy that focuses on your interpersonal skills and relationships. The therapist is verbal and directive, exploring interpersonal relationships in the past and present. The focus is on reducing symptoms, such as intense feelings of anxiety and depression that are exacerbated by these relationships. Interpersonal therapy has been shown to be effective with patients who are depressed.[7]

Marriage and family therapy looks at the family system and how all the elements work together (or don't work together), focusing not just on the individuals in the group but the functionality of the entire group as a whole. The therapist facilitates the process, which tends to be geared towards problem solving, boundary clarification, and identification of roles.

Group therapy typically involves a small group of people who have something in common such as their ages, the issues they face, or their therapeutic goals. The focus of these groups is usually relationship building, enhancing communication, boundary identification, support, and/or problem solving. The therapist is a facilitator.

Source: National Institute of Mental Health

types of therapies by going to the library, talking with family and friends, or getting on the Internet and exploring your options. Before you call a therapist, develop a list of questions that you want to ask, or use the sample questions provided on page 49 as a guide.

To find a therapist:

- Ask your doctor or clergy for a referral.
- Call a community mental-health center. These centers usually accept Medicaid and Medicare, and can bill you for treatment on a sliding scale.
- Check your health insurance or HMO's provider directory. Make sure whomever you choose accepts and is covered by your plan.
- Contact your employee assistance program.
- Call hotlines and crisis centers.
- Ask your friends and relatives.
- If you have financial concerns, look into community-based agencies, such as Jewish Family Services or Catholic Services. Such agencies can help people with mental-health issues at a significantly lower cost.
- Explore some of the resources in the Resources section under Mental Health, Marriage and Family.

What are you looking for? First of all, you're looking for a good fit. You have to feel comfortable with the therapist. You'll be sharing your feelings and personal information with this person. You don't want to feel as if you're being judged or criticized. The therapist should be a good listener.

> *Right after my heart attack, I was terribly fearful of everything and convinced that I would die of heart disease at a young age. I saw a therapist, and a psychiatrist in her group prescribed an antianxiety drug. Kathy [the therapist] listened to my fears—and she responded to me, too. I think she was eclectic in her approach. She gave me ideas to think about and solutions to problems I raised. At one point, she was trying very hard to convince me that not every problem would turn out to the worst possible end. I remember her using the example of a car accident that her son had*

---

7. Kemp et al, "Heart Disease."

at the time. The car was damaged in the accident, but her son was okay. She was trying to illustrate that something bad might happen but that the degree of damage or harm was variable, and one doesn't always have to assume the worst. I can't explain it, but that example has always stayed with me and whenever I hear of some terrible event, I try not to assume the worst and keep myself open for other possibilities. Sometimes I succeed. This serves me well with my heart disease.

—Irene, Springfield, NJ, age 51

With therapy, after a few months, you should begin to feel some relief and notice changes in your mood, behavior, and attitude. Be open with your therapist about how you're feeling and your progress. Your therapist should be receptive to your comments and concerns. You should feel absolutely comfortable being honest with your therapist. If for any reason you feel uncomfortable, you should share these thoughts with your therapist during your visits. If you think you are not getting the results you need, it may be that your therapist and the treatment you're receiving is not a good fit. But before making a change, discuss it with your therapist as part of the treatment process.

MEDICATION

I was warned that depression might happen. I was going to fight it. It arrived all of a sudden, without warning. After I tried to stay busy, I gave up and visited my internist. We talked about it and decided that the best idea was an antidepressant. I continue to be on some medication. My ability to cope is much better and I don't have the anxiety that I had right after the diagnosis. The dark pit was hell.

—Diana, Des Moines, IA, age 55

Medications can be life altering, especially for moderate to severe depression. Many studies tell us that psychotherapeutic medication helps women manage not only their anxiety and depression, but also their heart disease. These medications can improve mood and the quality of day-to-day life. They make it easier to stick with the heart medications and lifestyle changes that are essential to a healthy recovery. And ultimately, psychotherapeutic medications make it more likely that a patient with symptoms of depression or anxiety will survive and thrive. If you think about it, we are lucky that there are so many medications available to heart patients today that alleviate anxiety and depression, and that don't have negative interactions with our cardiovascular medications. At this writing, there's a study underway to determine whether both pharmacological and cognitive-behavioral therapy treatments will actually prevent a heart patient from experiencing another heart event.

Of course, to get medications, you have to first see a doctor. Many types of doctors feel comfortable prescribing medications for anxiety and depression. Medical doctors are the only professionals who can prescribe medication—your cardiologist, your internist, your ob-gyn, a psychiatrist,

INTERVIEWING A THERAPIST: WHAT TO ASK

1. What is your training? And what are your qualifications?
2. Are you licensed? Certified?
3. What treatment modality do you use in your practice?
4. What theoretical approach do you use in your treatment?
5. What is the average time you work with a patient or client?
6. How much experience do you have in treating this sort of problem?
7. Have you ever worked with a female heart patient?
8. How often do you treat women?
9. What do you charge?
10. Do you accept insurance?
11. What are your payment arrangements? Do you have a sliding scale fee?
12. What other types of therapy besides individual therapies do you offer?

The interview process helps you get the information you need to make an appropriate choice. As a practicing psychotherapist, I always appreciated clients who called to interview me about the way I conduct therapy. It gave me information about the client and told me that they were taking charge of their own care. You'll also want to check your insurance coverage to make sure that the therapist is covered, so the out-of-pocket expense is not too great. And always be sure your therapist is licensed and/or certified by the state in which you live.

or a medical psychiatrist. The best possible approach is to find a medical psychiatrist—that is, a psychiatrist who treats patients who have both medical and mental-health problems. Ideally, you'll want someone who is familiar with and experienced in treating women with heart disease. A medical psychiatrist should have the necessary knowledge of drug interactions and possible physical consequences or side effects.

To find a medical psychiatrist:

- Ask your internist, family practitioner, ob-gyn, health clinic, or cardiologist for a referral.
- Contact local medical and psychiatric societies.
- Go to the Yellow Pages and check under social services, counselors, mental-health services, psychologists, crisis hotlines, and physicians—psychiatry. They can give you a referral.
- Call your health insurance carrier or HMO.
- Inquire at community mental-health clinics or centers.
- Contact your Employee Assistance program.
- Get recommendations from family and friends.
- If you know a counselor, clinical social worker, licensed therapist, or psychologist, ask for a referral to a medical psychiatrist.
- Contact the American Psychiatric Association at 888-357-7924 to locate a psychiatrist near you.
- Contact the nearest University Medical Center to get a referral, or get on the Internet and access their faculty information.
- For further information, see the Resources section.

It is critical to make an informed decision. Feel free to interview a medical psychiatrist before you begin working with him or her. Ask questions. Have you treated women heart patients? What have you found successful for specific conditions? What kinds of complications or side effects might occur with certain medications? Do you recommend psychotherapy in conjunction with medication? And do you offer psychotherapy? Find someone that makes you feel comfortable, someone you feel you can trust. After what we've been through, we need doctors who will listen carefully and tailor their treatments to meet our needs—and medical psychiatrists are no exception.

When a medication is prescribed, you'll want to know:

- What types of foods or other medications should I avoid while I'm on these medications?
- How safe is it to drink alcohol with these medications?
- How long do I need to take medication?
- What are the possible drug interactions with heart medications?
- What happens when I get off these medications?
- If you're also seeing a psychotherapist, be sure to ask: How often will you communicate with my therapist and will you tell me when you do?

WHAT HEART PATIENTS SHOULD KNOW ABOUT MEDICATIONS FOR DEPRESSION AND ANXIETY

- Antidepressants are effective, but every woman is different as far as how she will tolerate the medication and how safe the medication is for her to take.
- The interactions between your cardiac medication and your medications for depression need to be closely monitored and reviewed by your doctor.
- SSRIs (selective serotonin reuptake inhibitors) seem to create fewer side effects and problems for patients with cardiovascular concerns. However, there can still be side effects even with these medications, so a physician needs to closely monitor you.
- If the SSRIs do not work effectively, there are still other medications that can be tried. Don't give up. Talk with your doctor.
- If you have an anxiety disorder, certain medications must be avoided due to your cardiac condition. A doctor can accurately assess this.
- Anxiety disorders can be treated effectively with many different kinds of medication. They include SSRIs, tricyclic antidepressants, benzodiazepines, beta-blockers, and monoamine oxidase inhibitors. Some of these medications might need to be avoided with certain types of cardiac problems and conditions.
- Be assertive and honest with your physicians about both your anxiety disorder and your cardiac condition.

If a doctor prescribes medication for you, don't expect immediate results. Every woman is different in how she will respond to treatment. Patience, along with clear and open communication with the doctor about how you are feeling, is particularly important in this phase. Here are a few things to keep in mind:

- Once you begin a medication, you might feel relief immediately or it might take several weeks to work, or sometimes longer.
- The dosage and types of medications may have to be adjusted.
- Never stop any medication without consulting with a doctor first. It can be unsafe to stop medications abruptly.
- Make sure your doctor knows all the prescription medications and over-the-counter medications you are taking.
- The amount of time you are on medications will depend on your individual needs, how well your symptoms have subsided, and whether your treatment goals have been reached.
- If you stop taking your medications, know that some of your symptoms may reoccur. Depending on your individual needs, you may need to stay on medication for a longer period of time.

JOIN A SUPPORT NETWORK

> [It's important] that every woman dealing with heart disease get support from someone who is knowledgeable, who has "been there." Breaking the bonds of isolation and shame at having heart disease is huge to coping and surviving heart disease.
>
> —Betty, Zanesville, OH, age 58

No matter what kind of therapy you seek, there is nothing that gives more relief than knowing that you are not alone. WomenHeart is the only advocacy organization in the country that serves this purpose through grassroots support networks, online community support and education, and community education and outreach. It is empowering to meet others who are heart patients like us. These are women who are willing to support us, listen to our stories without judgment, and talk to us with empathy—women who are actively doing something about heart disease.

I encourage you to visit the WomenHeart Web site at http://www
.womenheart.org/city_support_network.asp to locate support networks in
your area, communicate with other heart patients online, and take advantage of the educational resources. Or visit the American Self-Help Group
Clearinghouse, online at http://www.selfhelpgroups.org, for information
on support groups and other resources in your area. (See the Resources
section at the back of this book for more options.)

MOVING AHEAD

This chapter has given you tools to use to get the help you need. Once
you've found your emotional balance, it becomes easier to follow your
doctor's orders. All heart patients have to pay attention and manage their
risk factors. Chapter 4 will address ways you can change your thinking
and behavior to follow your doctor's orders without feeling deprived. I'll
show you ways to find that middle ground where restrictions don't rule
your life, and help you find healthy ways to reward yourself.

chapter four

FOLLOWING YOUR DOCTOR'S ORDERS

Those Pesky Risk Factors

Everything had to change. I had to face, accept, and then walk away from the many things that had brought me into this world of heart disease. I had to walk away from friendships that I realized were not emotionally healing to me. I had to walk away from a job that I loved for twenty years because I couldn't do it without pushing myself to an emotional breaking point. And the toughest was I had to run away from the diet pills, diets, and cigarettes that kept me going every day.
—Tasha, Hot Springs, AR, age 40

Tasha's heart event sent her a loud and important message. She knew she had to change her lifestyle choices. She also realized she could dramatically affect the future outcome of her health, improve the overall quality of her life, and improve her life expectancy by effectively managing her risk factors. Risk factor management is important in improving any woman heart patient's overall health and recovery. That's easily said, but it's one of the most difficult challenges that a woman heart patient faces. Just thinking about addressing issues related to your cholesterol, blood pressure, diabetes, weight, family history, age, smoking, or sedentary lifestyle can feel overwhelming. In response to all these new demands, it's difficult to know where to begin.

At first glance, it may seem easier just to avoid doing anything at all about changing your lifestyle. But we all know avoidance isn't healthy and that, in the long run, it will just cause more health problems. And deep down you know you can't afford to ignore your risk factors and tempt fate. So just try to take it one step at a time, as you would with anything that feels overwhelming.

THINK DIFFERENTLY ABOUT HEART DISEASE

I feel lucky to be here and to have been given the chance to live longer. I guess because my father had the "Hollywood Heart Attack" and didn't survive, I thought the survival chances weren't good. Not only did I survive but now there isn't much I feel I can't do. I can face just about anything now because I've faced, overcome, and moved on, while living well every day with heart disease.

—Diana, Des Moines, IA, age 55

It's easy to come home from the hospital thinking the worst. After all, you've been told you've got heart disease. The word "disease" in itself sounds scary—like an illness that's progressive, like something that will get worse over time. It also sounds permanent and, possibly, deadly. For starters, it's important that your image of heart disease changes. In truth, in most cases, heart disease is reversible. It doesn't have to be permanent or progressive. The reality is that you have tremendous control over your destiny with heart disease by choosing to actively reduce your risk factors.

MOVE FROM AWARENESS TO ACTION

Right now there are eight million women living in the United States with heart disease. In ten years, given the aging of the baby boom generation, it's predicted that more than 12 million women will be living with heart disease in the United States.[1] The good news is that most women in the United States now know that heart disease is the number one health risk

---

1. A ten-year population projection based on Census Bureau estimates calculated from NHLBI stats showing that 25% of women over 65 and 10% of women ages 45–64 have heart disease.

they face. Even so, there is a definite disconnect between awareness and action. Only a small percentage of those same women claim that they are personally at risk to get heart disease.[23] Just because you already have heart disease doesn't make it any easier to move from awareness to action. But if you've been diagnosed with heart disease, you've received a pretty loud wake-up call.

To move forward, you first need to recognize that these risk factors represent things that are within your control. Knowing your risk factors can help prevent future problems and empower you to change. So try to have a positive, optimistic attitude. That will go a long way toward en-abling you to take charge and do something about your heart disease—and to change your destiny. But where do you begin?

Begin by assessing where you are with your risk factors. Refer to the list on page 58, and determine which risk factors you have and what you know about them. For example, do you know your numbers for choles-terol and blood pressure? Are they too high? If you are a diabetic, is your blood sugar controlled? If you are someone who has to address multiple risk factors to improve your overall heart health, think about which fac-tors need to be addressed immediately. Speak to your health-care profes-sional. That can be a tremendous help in wading through the problem-solving process.

Then identify the risk factor you want to deal with first. Take on one risk factor at a time, and try this approach:

- First, come up with and write down reasons to attack that risk factor.
- Then brainstorm ideas of ways to reduce that personal risk fac-tor. Write down the list of ideas that you come up with.
- Then prioritize those ideas to come up with a list of your per-sonal goals for attacking that risk factor.

2. L. Mosca, W. K. Jones, K. B. King, et al., "Awareness, Perception, and Knowledge of Heart Disease Risk and Prevention among Women in the United States," *Archives of Family Medicine* 9, 2000: 506–15.

3. L. Mosca, H. Mochari, A. Christian, K. Berra, et al., "National Study of Women's Awareness, Preventive Action and Barriers to Cardiovascular Health," *Circulation* 113 (2006): 525–34.

Once you feel you have a plan for attacking your first risk factor, you can move on to the next, repeating those same steps. You'll find that some methods to reduce your risk factors will overlap—and that's a good thing. When that happens, life feels a bit less overwhelming. Here are some things to remember as you go through the process:

- Set goals that are clear, realistic, manageable, and achievable.
- Set a time frame to achieve your goals and adjust it as necessary.
- No matter what, do not give up! Even if you fall back into old habits, that's normal. Just get up the next day and start again.

RISK FACTORS

Even though you already have heart disease, it is still important to know your risk factors. Some of these risk factors are within your control. Others aren't. Either way, it's important for you to take steps to make changes in your lifestyle to improve your overall health outcome. Any of the following factors put a woman at risk for heart disease:

- Age fifty-five or older, and postmenopausal
- High blood pressure (140/90 or higher)
- High total cholesterol (over 200 mg/dL)
- Smoking
- Diabetes
- A family history of premature heart disease. That is, if your father or a brother was diagnosed with heart disease when he was younger than fifty-five; or your mother or sister was diagnosed at sixty-five or younger.
- Overweight by twenty pounds or more
- A sedentary lifestyle
- An unhealthy diet that's high in saturated fat, trans fat, cholesterol, and sodium; and low in fruits, vegetables, and fiber
- African American, Native American, or Hispanic

For more detailed information on risk factors consult your health-care provider and see the Resources and the Recommended Reading section in the back of this book.

A Step-by-Step Action Plan for Quitting Smoking

As an example, let's say your top priority risk factor is smoking. Your action plan might look something like this:

Step One: Come up with reasons to attack that risk factor, and write them down.

- Smoking is the number one preventable cause of death in the United States.
- It affects my health and dramatically increases my risk for many diseases, not just heart disease.
- It makes my clothes, car, house, breath, and body smell.
- It turns my teeth yellow and gives me wrinkles.
- It affects my breathing and my ability to do exercise.
- My kids hate it—and they're more likely to smoke if I smoke.
- I've seen my own father die from smoking.
- Socially, I have to find friends who are okay with smoking and that's not easy.
- It's inconvenient to smoke.
- I can save thousands of dollars a year that I spend on cigarettes.
- If I stop smoking for one year, I can cut my risk for further heart problems in half. And after several years of not smoking I will have no more risk of having more heart problems than someone who has not smoked. Now that's a good investment.

Step Two: Come up with some ideas to help you quit smoking.

- I can go to my doctor and pharmacist to get medications or stop-smoking aids (prescription and nonprescription), and have him/her give me suggestions on how to quit.
- I can go to a smoking-cessation program like SmokeEnders or Nicotine Anonymous. These programs can be found at

> *Heart disease due to blocked arteries is reversible through a process called arterial remodeling. Remodeling occurs when the damaging factors— smoking, cholesterol, high blood pressure—are controlled and the body can clear out the plaque. Women appear to be particularly good at remodeling, perhaps because their female hormones facilitate the repair processes. This may be a reason why women outlive men.*
>
> —Noel Bairey Merz, MD,
> Medical Director and Endowed Chair,
> Women's Health and
> Preventive Cardiology,
> Cedars-Sinai Medical Center

local hospitals, community centers, or through the human resources department at work. Or I can call the American Lung Association at (800) 242-8721 or the American Cancer Society at (800) 227-2345 for information.

- A combination approach may work best. I could get medication, go to a smoking cessation program, and get behavioral therapy as well.
- I can go to a therapist who uses hypnosis or explore the possibility of seeing an acupuncturist.
- I can start an exercise program first, so I'm less likely to gain weight when I stop smoking.
- I can start to cut down the number of cigarettes I smoke each day while I'm looking into these options.

Step Three: Set clear goals, including a time frame.

- I'll make an appointment to see my doctor and discuss the subject with him/her. I will call the doctor by the end of this week.
- I will also look into smoking cessation programs. I'll begin my research on Tuesday.
- I will start to exercise so that I don't gain too much weight when I quit smoking, by walking thirty minutes a day. Starting today!
- I will begin to cut down the number of cigarettes I smoke each day by only smoking outside the house. Starting today!
- My goal is to decide on a method of quitting smoking within the next three weeks, to begin the program by the end of the month, and to quit smoking completely by summer.

The good news is there are three ways that you can immediately begin to attack multiple risk factors at the same time. That's through diet, exercise, and taking your prescribed medications (see Medication Management in Chapter 1).

DIET NOT DRUDGERY

What it lies in our power to do, it lies in our power not to do.
—Aristotle

Your diet can effectively help control almost all risk factors. That's a powerful statement isn't it? But it doesn't make the prospect of following a heart-healthy diet any less overwhelming.

Let me take you back to your hospital experience for a second. Remember this? You're in the hospital after your heart event and a dietician comes into your room. She very politely tells you that you are overweight based on the body mass index, and that you'll have to change your diet to reverse your heart disease. Ultimately your new diet will play a big role in saving your life. She puts you on a 1,500-calorie diet, tells you to eat small meals and to choose from important food groups. She also tells you to watch out for saturated fats, trans fats, cholesterol, and sodium, among other things. From now on, she says, you're going to have to read labels and pay attention to the nutrient content of processed foods, many of which are high in sodium (salt) and sugar, as well as saturated fat and trans fat. She informs you that you need to eat foods with omega–3 fatty acids, and monounsaturated and polyunsaturated fats. But here's the good news: She says you can eat all of the fruits and vegetables you want. Yippee. I was thrilled, weren't you? You can also eat certain types of nuts—but only a handful per day.

She may tell you to eliminate caffeine from your diet or to reduce your caffeine intake. Then she tells you to switch from butter, margarine, lard, and shortening with trans fat to liquid vegetable oils such as olive, canola, soybean, sunflower, safflower, corn, or peanut oils. Red meat is okay sometimes, but you have to eat the extra-lean type. And it's important to control serving size; she advises a two- to three-ounce portion. That's about the size of a deck of playing cards. In fact, you need to cut the portions of just about everything you eat by half—except, of course, your fruits and vegetables. That's where you can really splurge. But there's more good news: You can drink a glass of wine every day. At this point, I'm thinking, only one?

If you were a bit overwhelmed, confused, even immobilized, by this visit from your dietician, you're not alone. I know I was.

Of course, the dietician is doing her job and doing it well. But after that little presentation the typical heart patient wants to hide somewhere and never come out again. You know that your diet can be better, that you can lose a little weight and that you're your own worst enemy. But when that health-care professional is in your hospital room, it forces you to confront a new reality and it seems like an awful lot to swallow.

Then you think about your family—your partner and children's eating habits—and the doubts become monumental. I, for one, just couldn't visualize my fussy eaters demolishing those fruits and vegetables with wild abandon. And I couldn't help but wonder when I was going to find the time and energy to do all the planning, shopping, cooking, and label reading such a diet would involve.

Okay, this is where you need to take a deep breath and realize that not all of these changes have to take place at once. It would be great if we could all change our diets immediately but, for most of us, that's unrealistic and unlikely.

Begin by taking small, incremental steps.   For example, start baking or grilling your foods instead of frying them. Use a nonstick pan, cooking spray, and liquid vegetable oils rather than butter, shortening, or lard for cooking and baking. Those are simple changes you can make immediately that will give you a long-term return on your short-term investment.

Remember it took you years to establish the eating habits you and your family have now. Giving yourself and your family time helps make the transition easier and more realistic. Start buying more fresh fruits and cutting back on processed foods. And start talking about the benefits of healthy eating.

Change is not always easy, but it can be done.   That's what I've learned from my five years of experience. I've also learned that heart-healthy foods can be delicious and acceptable to even your fussiest eaters. Explain to your family that there will be some changes in the foods at your house. Initially, there may be some resistance, but if you have a positive attitude and make the shift a gradual one, eventually everyone in your family will realize that good nutrition is for everyone's benefit—not just yours. In fact, adapting to a new diet can make the whole family feel connected to one another during a difficult time—and supportive of you.

My husband took on more responsibilities for the kids and home. He learned to cook heart-healthy meals "a la Dean Ornish" and often the whole family ate the same vegetarian dinners that I did.
—Irene, Springfield, NJ, age 51

If you need to lose weight, skip the fad diets. Fad diets may enable you to lose weight relatively quickly and even lower your cholesterol. But nutritionists agree that once you stop the diet—and start eating whatever was restricted on the diet—you'll put the weight right back on. And it may even create other health problems.

So what's the key to losing weight? I'm sorry to disappoint you but there's no magic pill or magic diet. My father and husband are both physicians and are so logical. Their secret to weight loss is simple: You must burn more calories than you consume each day. End of story. So if you have a less active day physically, you must eat fewer calories to lose or maintain your weight. And if you're physically more rigorous, you can eat more calories. Sounds simple, right?

KEEP IT SIMPLE

According to Penny Kris-Etherton, PhD, RD, Distinguished Professor of Nutrition at Pennsylvania State University, and an expert in cardiovascular nutrition, good nutrition practices are the cornerstone for the prevention and treatment of heart disease. A healthy diet will help control blood pressure and blood cholesterol levels—that is, reduce LDL cholesterol (the bad cholesterol). High blood pressure and high blood cholesterol levels are two significant risk factors for heart disease.

Dr. Kris-Etherton offers these manageable nutritional guidelines for heart patients:

- *Avoid certain fats.* The recommended diet for heart health is low in saturated fats, trans fat, and dietary cholesterol. Major sources of saturated fats are fatty red meats and full-fat dairy products. Lean meats, fish, and poultry and low-fat/fat-free dairy products are recommended. Commercially prepared desserts and snack foods (cakes, cookies, pastries, crackers, and chips) and deep-fried foods (french fries, fried chicken and fish, and onion rings) are major sources of trans fats. So you need to avoid them.
- *Reduce your sodium intake.* Choose and prepare foods with little salt. That means reading the labels of foods you cook with or eat. Commercially prepared foods are a major source of salt.
- *Eat a healthy mix of foods.* A healthy diet meets nutrient needs and provides adequate vitamins, minerals, and dietary fiber. Dietary guidance recommends consumption of:

  ○ 8–10 fruits and vegetables per day
  ○ 3 servings of whole grains per day

WATCH YOUR PORTIONS

Twenty years ago, the average portion of spaghetti and meatballs was one cup. With three meatballs, that's about 500 calories. Today, the average portion of spaghetti is two cups, which, with three meatballs, equals 1,025 calories. That's twice the calories!

- *Watch serving sizes.* A healthy serving of most foods is about the size of a tennis ball or a deck of cards—that is, much smaller than most people realize.
- *Check product labels.* Get in the habit of checking product labels to determine calorie counts per serving—and the number of servings per package or container.
- *Find out more.* For more information on portion sizes—and to see how much additional physical activity is needed to burn the extra calories that come with these larger portions—visit http://hp2010.nhlbihin.net/portion.

    °   3 servings of low-fat/fat-free dairy products per day
    °   Fish, especially high in omega-3 fatty acids (fatty fish such as salmon, tuna, and trout). Two servings of fish per week are recommended.

- *Control portion size.* Weight control is very important for heart health. Because portion size has increased dramatically over the years, it's essential to be aware of this and control portion size as a way to control calories and achieve a healthy body weight.

THE BARRIERS TO BETTER EATING

If it's so logical and simple, why isn't it easy to follow healthy eating guidelines? Why is it so hard to eat right? Why is change so difficult? First of all, I said it was logical—I didn't say it was easy. Every day, many women wage an emotional battle against themselves in trying to change the way they eat. Our eating habits are deeply ingrained, and when you try to change those patterns, you have to give something up. It feels like a loss. Here are the reasons I've heard over and over: I don't want to feel deprived; I don't want to be told what to do; I can't accept that I'm growing older and that this is a necessity; I don't want to think of myself as having no choice because I've got heart disease; I've been like this forever and can't change—I'm too far gone; I don't know where to start.

These old patterns of thinking and behavior are connected to something meaningful to you—somehow you've invested in your eating habits. Maybe you feel a sense of security about how and what you eat or a sense of control. Letting someone else tell you what to put in your mouth and buying into the whole healthy eating routine means, essentially, giving up some control. In addition, certain foods may give you tremendous pleasure, maybe the only pleasure you experience during the day.

As it is, having heart disease feels as if you've lost some control over your body—your body and heart let you down by getting ill. And you can no longer do whatever you want to do. *I know it's not fair.* These feelings of anger and sadness coupled with the fact that being on a diet feels like physical deprivation can set you up to not change and keep you stuck. Rebelliousness is a common reaction.

This resistance to change *for your own good* may be rooted in your personal history and your psychology. Your early experiences and influences can still have an effect on your behavior and thinking today. Look inside and think hard about how you use food daily. What does food do for you? Here are some questions you might ask yourself:

- Do you eat out of boredom, frustration, or anxiety?
- Do you use food to soothe and comfort you, or to relieve emotional distress?
- Does your thinking about food go to extremes—it's either all or nothing.
- Are you a person who thinks of foods as good or bad, and that you have to be a perfect dieter or forget it?

If you have these kinds of issues around food, it's possible that you'll sabotage your good intentions and have trouble changing the way you eat. If you tend to use food to relieve anxiety or emotional distress, a vicious cycle can develop. Food can bring you immediate relief and satisfaction, but later cause more distress. If you're a diet perfectionist, a minor slipup can result in self-sabotage, and feelings of guilt and shame. You'll want to break these patterns so you don't undermine your efforts. If you're struggling with these kinds of issues, don't hesitate to consult your doctor or nutritionist for guidance. They may recommend therapy, counseling, or a support group in your area.

Believe it or not, for many heart patients, changing deeply ingrained eating habits is one of the toughest challenges of all. But ultimately it will be the most meaningful and long lasting. I promise, over time, the way you think and feel about food will change.

The first and hardest step for every heart patient is acceptance—simply acknowledging that if you want to thrive, you're going to have to change, that there's no shortcut; and that a heart-healthy diet is essential if you're going to improve your health and live your life to the fullest. Once that realization takes hold, you can begin to think of food as one of your most valuable allies—as a weapon in the battle for better health rather than your enemy. You'll find that being on a heart-healthy diet actually gives you tremendous control—the control to influence your health for the rest of your life. You'll also become a positive role model and influence those you care about by making these changes. And that's a pretty powerful reason to change!

FIFTEEN WAYS TO AVOID SELF-SABOTAGING

Develop a plan for your diet and then smell the roses and enjoy each day.

—Judy, Kenai, AK, age 63

1. *Break the emotional link.* Recognize that eating may be connected to your emotional state, that you may be using food to comfort yourself. That's a habit you'll want to break. Try to anticipate and identify those high-risk emotional situations where food seems to be giving you the quickest relief. When these situations arise, plan for alternatives that will help you to deal with your emotions. For example, instead of eating, you can take a walk, write in a journal, paint a picture, work in your garden, take a nap, read a book, or talk to a friend or family member. Try not to eat away your frustration, anger, sadness, or other feelings. Remember, if you're eating to make yourself feel better, it may work in the short run, but not in the long run. In fact, you may feel bad about it in just a few hours.

2. *Monitor yourself.* Pay attention to what you are eating and how much. If you eat in front of the television, movies, or while reading, you'll likely be distracted and not focus on your food intake. Clearly, when distracted we eat more of the foods that are wrong for us and we eat more than we would normally. Just think about all the unhealthy food we consume at the movies. That says it all!

3. *Think positively.* Remember the "D" in diet is not for drudgery or deprivation; this is going to be a positive lifestyle change that lasts the rest of your life. It will take some time, so be patient. Think of your new heart-healthy diet as a rewarding commitment to your future health. Embrace these changes as positive and be proud with each new success. As you begin to see and feel the results of your efforts, your energy will improve, you'll be less tired, and you'll feel better.

4.   *Get some help.* Talk to a health-care professional, nutritionist, or dietician about an appropriate diet for you. They can clarify and spell out the portion sizes, and help you create a balanced heart-healthy diet that's best for you. They can also help you weed through the myths and misconceptions of the many diets that are promoted today and explain which ones to avoid. There may be some foods you refuse to give up. Explain your reasons to your health-care professional or dietician and work out a compromise.

5.   *Moderation is the key.* My grandmother was ninety-two years old when she died. She was one of the wisest women I knew and she'd had a bypass in her early sixties. When I asked her at ninety-one years old how she kept so thin and healthy, her response was, "Moderation is the key to eating and living." She advised: "Drink lots of water and avoid as many processed foods as possible." Logical, isn't she?

6.   *Don't judge yourself.* Try not to view your eating habits as good or bad. Or view your daily food intake as a black or white issue. That just sets you up to fail, because it leads to feelings of guilt or deprivation. Being perfect with your diet is not the goal. Reversing and managing your heart disease is the goal.

7.   *Start slowly with your diet and take small steps.* Realize most women have been eating without consciously thinking about it since childhood. Just be consistent and persistent in your eating habits. If you have a bad day where you eat a donut or a piece of fried chicken or a double helping of pasta, don't give up. Forgive yourself and go back to your healthy eating habits the next day. Give yourself a break mentally. Women are so good at beating themselves up for making mistakes. Trying daily to improve your eating habits is what's important. Remember nobody's perfect all of the time!

8.   *Try writing in a food journal.* Journals help document what you are really eating. Studies show that when people guess their daily calorie and fat intake, they are off by a significant amount, which actually can result in weight gain.[4]

---

4. M. A. Zegman, "Errors in Food Recording and Calorie Estimation: Clinical and Theoretical Implications for Obesity," *Addictive Behaviors* 9 (4) 1984: 347–50.

EATING RIGHT AND GAINING WEIGHT?

Be aware that you can gain weight on a heart-healthy diet—like I did. My heart may have been happier but my clothes didn't fit as well. What can you do? Just continue to be conscientious about the number of calories you're consuming each day. I later learned that I needed to eat between meals to prevent myself from getting too hungry and then overeating at the next meal. A dietician helped me to figure out what to eat during those important snacking times, which helped me greatly and I lost the weight I had gained.

Work with your dietician or nutritionist to figure out how many calories you can consume each day to lose or maintain your weight. And, again, be sure you have access to a health professional who can help you map out your diet, and help you when questions arise. If your doctor doesn't offer to refer you to a dietician or nutritionist, be assertive and ask for a referral.

9.   *Read labels.* Train yourself to read labels. It really helps to identify portion sizes, calories, fat content, salt, and cholesterol in the products you are buying.

10.   *Avoid fast food.* Most Americans have grown up on fast food and learned that if they don't "super size" their food they are being deprived or, worse still, wasting money. It's a matter of changing your mindset and recognizing most of the food at these establishments is just not good for you. The next time you're in a fast-food restaurant, ask for a nutrition guide that shows the calories and fat content in each of the foods they serve. You'll be shocked!

11.   *Shop the periphery.* Kathy Smith, one of the premier exercise experts in the country, suggests that, when you're shopping at the grocery store, try to spend most of your time shopping around the edge of the store along the walls, instead of in the center aisles. That way, you'll load up on fruits, vegetables, protein, and whole grains rather than processed foods.

12.   *Take a day off.* Allow one day a week to be a cheat day, but don't go overboard. And there's nothing wrong with eating a small piece of dark chocolate every day. If that's your thing, it's actually heart healthy.

13. *If it's not there, you won't eat it.* Keep healthy foods in abundance in your house and limit junk food so that you have a healthy food environment at home. It's essential that kids learn good eating habits early. Nutritionists recommend not prohibiting certain foods but limiting them.

14. *Drink more water.* No matter what type of diet changes you make, it's critical to drink a lot of water. Some dieticians recommend at least eight full glasses of water daily. The water will keep you hydrated and make you feel full. It's also good for your gastrointestinal system. Your health-care provider will often tell you to drink a lot of water because of all the medications you're taking. And because you'll be eating more fiber, you'll need to drink more water to aid digestion.

15. *Think of food as fuel.* Think of your body as a train that needs the best fuel to run effectively and efficiently. Putting food in your

GET CREATIVE ABOUT FOOD

Create a buddy system through which you can share food and cooking tips, exchange information, and provide assistance.

—Mary, Cortlandt Manor, NY, age 54

Try to enjoy your new approach to food. Be creative. And take pleasure in it. Here are some ideas:

- Go to the farmer's market for your fruits and vegetables. Your kids will love it and it might motivate everyone to try to eat more fresh produce.
- Buy some heart-healthy cookbooks and magazines. (See the back of this book for some great resources.)
- Watch some cooking shows. And try out the recipes!
- Get on the Web and look for healthy recipes that appeal to you and your family.
- Create your own scrapbook of everyone's favorites.
- Tell your family that you're experimenting and that they are the guinea pigs. Nobody needs to know that the foods you are cooking are good for them. Shhh, it's our secret!

body should not cause you stress or guilt. The food you eat is just the fuel that all of us need to pump the engine!

EXERCISE: IT'S NOT A FOUR-LETTER WORD

If you find a path with no obstacles, it probably doesn't lead anywhere.

—Frank Clark, Athlete

Like a heart-healthy diet, regular exercise can have a significant impact on modifying any woman heart patient's risk factors. In Chapter 1, I talked about the importance of cardiac rehabilitation as a first step forward to improving your health and well-being. Beginning a regular exercise program is the next step in that process, and a crucial step in your journey. And, like healthy eating, exercise has its own set of rewards—and obstacles.

"Women with heart disease must actually overcome two mental obstacles as they begin their exercise program," says Tommy Gerber, a certified personal trainer and attorney. "The first is one faced by many people when they start exercising for the first time—the intimidation factor of coming into a new environment where they are probably not particularly comfortable in utilizing machines and/or exercises with which they're not familiar. The second is a bit more particular to heart patients: How hard can I work? Many heart patients don't get the full benefits of exercise, which they should enjoy, because they're afraid that working too hard will actually cause further heart problems."

If you're a person who has avoided exercise her entire life, it's even more important for you to begin to exercise every day. The Dietary Guidelines for Americans 2005 now recommend thirty minutes of moderate exercise a day for everyone—that's in addition to your normal activities.[5] If you start slow, follow your doctor's recommendations, and make a half hour a day your ultimate goal, you can change your weight and heart health for the rest of your life.

---

5. Dietary Guidelines for Americans 2005, published by the Department of Health and Human Services (HHS) and the Department of Agriculture (USDA), http://www.healthierus.gov/dietaryguidelines.

GET THAT HEART PUMPING

Exercise enables your heart to pump blood. Over time, that increases your tolerance for more exercise. And that, in turn, enhances your ability to participate in the activities of daily living—which improves the overall quality of your life. A regular exercise regimen:

- Helps with weight loss and maintenance.
- Reduces your heart rate.
- Decreases your tension, anxiety, and possibly stress.
- Improves your mood.
- Lessens fatigue.
- Improves your appearance, confidence, and how you feel about yourself.
- Improves your overall blood lipid and cholesterol profiles.
- Helps to decrease blood pressure for people with hypertension.
- Reduces your risk factors for developing other diseases such as cancer, diabetes, and even dementia.

Why is exercise so hard for many women?

As little girls, many of us were not encouraged to participate in sports. That was guy stuff. And, while most of us attended gym class, we did so only because we had to. Many of us dreaded it. While boys were encouraged—if not pushed—to do sports, most girls were discouraged. Athletic girls were labeled tomboys and even made fun of for these masculine pursuits. Of course, all that has changed today. Young women are encouraged to lead active, healthy, sports-filled lives. But that wasn't true in the 1950s and 1960s, and for many women over the age of fifty, exercise has played only a small role in their lives. So the first obstacle to exercising that most women face is their exercise history—or lack thereof. These women are unsure and insecure about where to start when it comes to exercise. Some are embarrassed to exercise in public and even more so if men are around.

Another obstacle to overall fitness in our society today relates to technology. Women are so plugged into their cell phones, blackberries, computers, and televisions that they've forgotten how to block out time to be away from all of these disturbances. I saw the funniest thing a few days ago: a woman out walking in sneakers and running clothes. She had a cell phone in one hand and a document in the other. And she was talking on the phone, reading, and walking at the same time. At least she was trying to get some exercise. It's amazing how many women still talk on their phones while working out on machines in the gym. Women, in particular, have allowed themselves to be too accessible to anyone who wants to reach them, anytime. Unplugging and disconnecting from the outer world seems to be a struggle for many. Trying to multitask every moment of the day seems to be the problem.

The ability to listen to your body and the overall fulfillment you get from exercise gets lost in all the noise. Many women don't even listen to their own breathing during exercise. Losing touch with your inner self and your body gives you little time to decompress, relax, and process feelings. And that's not good for you.

If you approach it without other distractions, exercise can be like a high, generating feelings similar to ones you might experience when meditating, enjoying sex, savoring a piece of dark chocolate, or watching a spectacular sunset. Exercise can give you that high because, as you exercise, neurohormones are released into your body that can produce intense feelings of joy and pleasure.

If you've never exercised before, how do you get started?

> *I was in a cardiac rehabilitation program and had bought a treadmill for the house. I considered daily exercise as important as taking my medications. To this day, I exercise an hour a day, usually six days a week. The treadmill is in the family room. My husband is usually on the computer, my youngest one hangs out watching TV, and I'm there for him, as needed.*
>
> —Irene, Springfield, NJ, age 51

Before having a heart event, you could make excuses for not exercising. Now you know that exercise will improve your overall health, longevity, and well-being. You can't put it off any longer. Like breathing and sleeping, exercise has to become part of your daily routine. I can hear the moans from here, but the truth is that if you want to change your health outcome dramatically, the one thing you have to do is exercise. Health-care professionals, personal trainers, and sports physiologists aren't try-ing to make you miserable, they're simply telling you the truth.

For Women Who Have Always Exercised: How Do You Get It Back?

> *Both of my very mild heart attacks came about eight hours after vigorous exercise—a thirteen-mile walk and a two-and-a-half-mile run. After that, I had several false restarts before I began walking regularly. I never liked walking. It felt like I was in an imaginary race behind my former, fitter self, trudging slowly, bringing up the rear. My stroll was a far cry from leading fitness classes or completing a three-day mountain bike ride. I wanted to ride but I wasn't sure I could trust my heart again.*
>
> —Nichele, Birmingham, AL, age 40

Like Nichele, you may be one of those women who has exercised a good portion of your life and then had a heart event, so you feel skeptical, hesitant, and scared to get back to exercising. Heart disease may have even reared its ugly head while you were exercising, as it did with me. This event might have left you feeling abandoned or betrayed by your own body. These feelings are normal.

The rules for you are the same as for those who have never exercised. The main difference is that you may think that after a heart event you'll get back physically to where you were before and will do so quickly. Well, the reality is that your body has been through a trauma and as with any trauma it will take time, patience, and healing to get back to where you were with exercise. But don't worry, over time it'll happen.

If you have any fears, speaking to your cardiologist can reassure you. But realize you might have to build up your strength at a slower rate than you'd prefer. Just like any woman who has had a heart event, you'll need to start slow and then build up your physical endurance, strength, and ability. Cardiac rehabilitation is a great beginning even for you. After cardiac rehabilitation you might want to consider getting a personal trainer to put you on a challenging but safe exercise routine. Typically, you can get referrals to trainers through your cardiac rehabilitation center. The trainer can put you on a heart rate monitor while you exercise for your safety as well as to know your physical strengths and limitations. Make sure the trainer has worked with heart patients before. That gives you extra peace of mind. If you find that you are immobilized and frustrated in getting back to exercise, you might want to find out what's going on. Deeper issues and fears may require therapy to help you begin to trust your body so you can enjoy exercising again. (See the Resources section and Chapter 3 for information on finding help when you need it.)

Eventually, you will find your way back to exercise. It may be a whole new program and a new way to exercise but you will find that those changes are for the better.

> *I had to find my own answers. I bought a spiffy red heart rate monitor. By staying within about 75 percent of my maximum heart rate, it reassured me and kept me focused on what was going on inside rather than how fast I was going or how many laps I was doing. I overcame the fear by going back beyond square one to square negative one, being gentler with myself, and moving slowly toward this "new normal" in which I'm stronger, fitter, and a bit wiser.*
>
> —Nichele, Birmingham, AL, age 40

WHERE TO BEGIN — WHATEVER YOUR EXERCISE HISTORY

First, talk to your doctor.   Before you begin any exercise program make sure you get guidance and permission from your physician. If you've been in cardiac rehabilitation, still speak to your doctor about starting a program on your own and what that program will entail.

Make a plan.   See below for information on how to begin an exercise regimen. Incorporate input from your doctor, your cardiac rehabilitation program, and a fitness professional, if at all possible.

Once you have a plan, just do it.   Don't think too much about it. Like the commercial says, just do it—or you'll find a way to talk yourself out of it. Striving for wellness is hard work and a commitment to yourself every day.

Schedule it in, daily.   Exercise should be one of the activities you do daily that's just for you. You need to set aside time every day. That may involve rearranging your schedule, whether that means eating dinner an hour later, getting your partner to drive the kids to school, or cutting back on your television time every day. You'll find this is one of the best changes you can make for yourself. It will refresh and rejuvenate you so you can do all of your other activities with vim and vigor.

Enlist your family's support.   According to fitness trainer Tommy Gerber, it's important to get your family on board before embarking on an exercise program. "I honestly believe just knowing your family is behind you and you're doing the right thing means a lot before you step on the treadmill for the first time," says Gerber.

Get some help from a trained professional.   "The other critical factor is to get some help from a trained professional who knows not only about the exercises you're contemplating, but how they affect your condition," says Gerber. "Even for those women who have exercised extensively prior to their diagnosis, this is important for both your own safety and for building your confidence."

How to Get Moving Again: Make a Plan

Where do you start? How much exercise is too much? How do you know it's safe? Well, if you started with cardiac rehabilitation, keep going. If you didn't, you can begin with something as simple as gardening, cleaning your house, or actively playing with your kids or dogs. But, again, talk to your doctor first and get permission before you start any physical activity. For starters, just move your body in space. That can mean simply walking around your house or your neighborhood. Those small steps feel great and will make you feel much better. Here are some more suggestions to get you moving:

- *Start small.* Start with a five- to ten-minute walk every day and add time as you become more conditioned. You can walk at a school track, a park, or your neighborhood.
- *Do what's natural.* Take your dog for a walk. Romp around with your kids. You can take your children to exercise with you at the park, on hiking trails, or at the swimming pool.
- *Use a pedometer.* Count your steps by using a pedometer. Shape Up America recommends that you try to build up to 10,000 steps per day. Go to www.shapeup.org for more information.
- *Join a gym or health club.* Take beginning classes at a gym to get into shape slowly but steadily. Gyms are always running specials to join and can be very reasonably priced. Another option is local YWCA/YMCA, which offer excellent classes, trainers, and weight and cardiovascular equipment.
- *Again, if you can afford a personal trainer, get one.* He/she can build your confidence and give you a preliminary routine you can start with and get you to a point where you'll feel comfortable with the equipment and moving your body.

IS IT SAFE?

The best way to overcome the initial fears regarding exercise is to take these important steps to ensure you're not overdoing it.

- Start with cardiac rehabilitation. That way, your first steps at exercise will be monitored. If your doctor doesn't refer you to cardiac rehab, be assertive: Ask for a referral.
- Get your doctor's permission before beginning any kind of exercise program.
- Always start slow and build up gradually, so your body can adjust.
- Monitor how you feel and act accordingly. If you feel odd in any way when you're exercising, contact your doctor and discuss those feelings. Don't be afraid to ask questions. (See Chapter 9 about how to talk to your doctor about these kinds of issues.)

- *Find an exercise buddy.* This can be critical in giving you cama- raderie, companionship, and competition. Sometimes having a friend who will both support and drive you will be the most mo- tivating factor and get you moving. That can mean simply taking a daily walk with a friend.
- *Get into a routine.* Be as consistent as possible and create a rou- tine, so that you're more apt to follow through with your plan. But that doesn't mean make it boring. You can develop a routine with the same people, at the same time, and at the same place but do different exercises to keep it interesting and fun!
- *It's a must-do.* Think of exercise as a "must" rather than a "should." Knowing that it's just part of your daily routine, like taking a shower, brushing your teeth, or taking your medica- tions, helps to put exercise and physical activity in the proper perspective.
- *Be creative.* Take advantage of any opportunity to move your body in space even if it just means taking the stairs instead of the elevator. As time goes by, you'll feel free to explore all kinds of exercise options—biking, yoga, belly dancing, Pilates—as long as you have your doctor's permission.

My mind is telling me not to exercise, now what?

After you start moving your body in space, there will be days when you'll wonder why you're making exercise a priority. Excuses can begin to creep into your thinking. You might tell yourself that you don't have enough time or energy and that you're getting bored with your exercise routine anyway. It's important to work through these momentary lapses and get back out there. Don't beat yourself up when you have these thoughts. Just get your tennis shoes on, stop thinking, and get out the door—or onto the treadmill. Strive to be the best that you can be by working toward realistic, attainable goals. Here are strategies to keep you going:

- *If you feel a lack of energy:* Tell yourself that exercise will reinvigo- rate you. But respect your body's time clock for exercise. Some times of day will be better for exercise than others. Exercise at the best time of day for your body. If you really are tired, do a less intensive workout or just go for a walk. Break down your exercise program and, for that day, go back to doing ten minutes of exercise. It's likely that once you get started, you'll find that you'll probably exercise for longer than you planned.

- *If you find you don't have time:* Reduce the time you spend on exercise—but keep in mind that thirty minutes is a small portion of your day. More and more gyms are instituting shorter exercise classes because so many people are crunched for time. The most important thing is just to stick with it. Exercising a shorter period of time is better than not exercising at all.
- *If you're bored:* Vary your exercise routine. Swim one day, work out in the gym the next, take a walk another day, take exercise classes or work out to a video. If you vary your exercise routine, boredom is less likely to cause you problems.

The last important statement I want to leave you with about exercise is one that I heard a radio announcer say one day: "The best exercise to get, is the exercise you do." That says it all!

EXPERT ADVICE ON EXERCISE

Here are some exercise tips directly from Kathy Smith, author of more than a dozen books on fitness and nutrition, including *Kathy Smith's Walkfit for a Better Body* and *Kathy Smith's Flex Appeal: Look Great and Feel Sexy at Any Age:*

It's normal for women to occasionally hit plateaus with their exercise routine. The body is very adaptable. A routine becomes just that within a few weeks: a routine. Your body will adapt to even the most perfect routine, rendering it ho-hum in even three weeks. Additionally, it's important to give the body different stimulations and stresses. By varying the stresses the body receives you will not only get more out of your workouts by stimulating a variety of muscles, you will also be at a lower risk for overuse injuries. Even the most talented runners will find that they run better and have fewer injuries if they cross-train and do different modes of cardio workouts during the week, like cycling or swimming.

HEART ATTACK WARNING SIGNS AND SYMPTOMS — AND WHAT TO DO

Exercise is critical to your recovery and your overall health. But when you begin an exercise program, it's important to know the warning signs of a potential heart attack:

- Discomfort, fullness, tightness, squeezing, or pressure in the center of the chest that stays for more than a few minutes or comes and goes.
- Pressure or pain that spreads to your upper back, shoulders, neck, jaw, or arms.
- Dizziness or nausea.
- Clammy sweats, heart flutters, or paleness.
- Unexplained feelings of anxiety, fatigue, or weakness—especially with exertion.
- Stomach or abdominal pain.
- Shortness of breath and difficulty breathing.

If you're having several of these heart attack warning signs, you need to take action immediately:

- Call 911 for an ambulance or have someone drive you to the nearest hospital emergency room immediately. Do not delay! Tell the hospital staff that you're having heart attack symptoms.
- Chew and swallow with water one regular full-strength aspirin as soon as possible to prevent blood clotting.
- Insist that the hospital staff take your complaints seriously, do not make you wait, and give you a thorough cardiac evaluation including an electrocardiogram (EKG) or an echocardiogram, and a blood test to check your cardiac enzymes.

Source: WomenHeart Web site at www.womenheart.org

Building variety into your workout week is very important. You might want to try yoga one day instead of your normal cardio workout. I recommend cardio exercise thirty to forty minutes a day, at least five to six days a week. There are myriad ways to achieve this.

- Vary your routine by exercising to a home exercise tape one day, doing a cycling or swimming workout the next, and so on.
- Add brisk-paced walking outside to help ease boredom.
- Find friends to exercise with. People who exercise with a workout buddy tend to have better adherence to their exercise consistency than those who exercise alone.
- Go to the gym to work out on the equipment or take a group exercise class. Most gyms have group cycling, strength training, Pilates mat classes, and a variety of cardio classes.
- Try to do a few days of resistance training every week and vary that experience too. Strength training is the fastest way to recapture lost muscle mass and reshape the body. Just two or three strength-training workouts spread out through the week is all you need.
- If you can afford it, hire a personal trainer for a few sessions to help motivate you, keep your routine fresh, and learn proper form and alignment.

But no matter what, don't stop exercising. Work through your feelings and keep moving! No exercise program can work its magic without consistency. Consistency is the key to results.

Looking Inward

A heart-healthy diet, an exercise plan, and strategies for addressing your risk factors and improving your overall health—that's a great beginning. In the next chapter, we'll turn our attention back to your inner self—how you feel about your body, your sense of mortality, your sexuality, and your self-image.

PART TWO

REBUILDING YOUR SENSE OF SELF

If wrinkles must be written upon our brows, let them not be written upon the heart. The spirit should never grow old.

—John Kenneth Galbraith

chapter five

BODY IMAGE AND THE SEXUAL SELF

Relaxation and Renewal

I am beautiful as I am.
I am the shape that was gifted.
My breasts are no longer perky and upright
like when I was a teenager.
My hips are wider than that of a fashion model.
For this I am glad, for these are
the signs of a life lived.

—Cindy Olsen, Actress

BODY IMAGE

Body image begins at birth. The way you are held, touched, loved, and nurtured from childhood through adolescence affects how you see yourself throughout your life. How was sex viewed and discussed in your home? Was your family open in addressing your curiosity about your own body—and other people's? Or were you made to feel ashamed, guilty, and fearful? How your family responded to you has a tremendous impact on your body image and your sexual self.

Adolescence is a tumultuous time. Teenagers are bombarded by messages from their families, the media, and their peers. Those messages affect the way they think and feel about their bodies as well as how they think others see them. For some adolescence is like being swept up in a hormonal tornado and then dropped in a world that's not unlike Oz—inside out and upside down. Believe me I know. I have three teenage sons and sometimes find myself in the center of the storm! How were sex and body issues handled by the adults around you when you were at this stage in your life? The experiences you had and the messages you received as a teenager influenced your self-confidence and self-esteem as an adult.

Fast forward to the childbearing years, when women begin to see changes in their bodies that reveal imperfections. Remember the first time you saw stretch marks or cellulite? Traumatic, wasn't it? Whether you had children or not, you probably began noticing physical changes during your twenties and thirties. Then, if you're like a lot of women, you started trying to modify these imperfections with diet, exercise, a makeover, or even, in extreme cases, plastic surgery. Today a surprising number of women in their twenties and thirties are preoccupied with trying to get their bodies to morph back to a younger state—and with trying to hold back the aging process.

Of course, as women approach midlife, it becomes harder and harder to attain that youthful ideal.

> *Old age ain't no place for sissies.*
> —Bette Davis

With the onset of middle age comes a whole new set of changes: the graying hair, the eyeglasses, those infernal wrinkles, and hairs that appear in places you never expected—on your breasts, your neck, your upper lip, your chin.

Gravity compounds the issue: Your breasts move south and your hips begin cruising east and west. Even the skin on your face heads southward. Round about the same time, you begin to notice that your ability to remember names, dates, and bits of trivia waxes and wanes, further enhancing your insecurities and self-doubt.

Of course, midlife means the onset of menopause, which can wreak havoc on your emotions and your body. During and following menopause, some women gain weight more easily and notice a thickening around their waists. Others experience mood swings, night sweats, and hot flashes, sometimes so severe that they believe everyone is watching them turn beet red as the sweat forms on their brows. It can be embarrassing and awkward. These physical changes can test a woman's self-image and self-confidence.

Through all these stages, it can be hard to ignore all of the messages society has been sending women for years—that youth is beauty and outward appearance is everything. Those messages can get in the way of our ability to develop an accurate self-perception and healthy body image. As a result, women are quick to judge themselves by their outer appearance—not the inner qualities that make each individual so special. We are socialized to believe that what's most important relates not to who we are, and how we feel and act and think, but to how we look—as measured against an unrealistic standard.

Americans are obsessed with physical beauty. The entertainment industry and the mass media embrace physical beauty as the ideal. We have magazines and entire television shows built around such subjects as "The Most Beautiful People of 2007" and "The World's Sexiest Women." And, boy, do subscriptions and ratings soar!

Women have been inundated since early childhood with messages about how they should look and dress, and, most importantly, what their bodies should look like. Often, it seems, the American ideal of a perfect woman is one with a young, flawless body, and that a woman's ultimate purpose—whether she's at work or at home raising kids, at the Laundromat or at her computer—is to be sexy. It's an ideal that bears little relationship to the lives most women live. And as we move into middle age, those messages test our self-esteem and positive self-image as it becomes harder and harder to attain that youthful ideal.

Given our culture's preoccupation with how young we should look and how outwardly sexy we're supposed to be, many women have unresolved internal conflicts about growing older. Thrust a life-threatening heart event on top of a woman's already fragile feelings about her physical self, and it can turn into a full-blown crisis, magnifying her negative feelings about herself and her body. For women heart patients already grappling with issues associated with aging, a heart event can intensify these conflicts. How do you deal with it? Believe it or not, this can be a powerful opportunity to get past all those unrealistic messages so that a new, healthier sense of self can emerge.

CHANGING YOUR THINKING:
HOW DO YOU TALK TO YOURSELF?

I'm going to a wedding in August and because I'm self-conscious, I'll be wearing a different design of dress than all of the other brides-maids to accommodate my scar. I hope to be as beautiful as them. I haven't worn formal attire since my bypass surgery. I'm so nervous!
—Sarah, West Hempstead, NY, age 29

You walk up to the mirror and, in your head, you're still a spry, young thing. But then your reflection stops you in your tracks. Who is that? you ask yourself. Is that me? Omigosh. I look like my mother! It's a completely normal reaction. You see that you're no longer that perky teen you still feel like on the inside. You see the changes in your body. You see the scars—and looking at your body can be difficult.

What do you say to yourself when you look at your reflection? Do you respond negatively? Are you hard on yourself? Or are you kind and gentle? Do you give yourself a compliment and a pat on the back, a reward for managing your life so well? The messages you send yourself—day after day—have an enormous impact on your outlook, attitude, body image, mood, and self-esteem.

So if you're feeling negative, how can you rearrange those feelings about yourself and point them in a positive direction?

Take good care of yourself.   It's important for you to nurture a healthy mental attitude toward the things that you can control about your body. That means eating right, exercising, pampering yourself (see page 93), and controlling stress (see pages 92–96). These are the surest ways to improve your overall body image and mental attitude. Focusing on what you can do to enhance your wellness and your happiness will make it much easier to cope with the aging process. And if you set a goal of being the healthiest you can be, that will help you refocus your energy more on the inside of your body than the outside.

When it comes to self-esteem, attitude really is everything. Reward yourself with praise instead of talking to yourself about what's missing or wrong with you. A wise woman once told me to stand tall with confidence when I walk and others will see me as a taller person inside and out. She was right. But sometimes you need to tell yourself these things every day to get it.

Think positively. How you think about yourself can change how you feel about yourself and your life in an amazing way. If you rethink your positive traits, you might find that there's more to you than you give yourself credit for. For example, in *Sex and the Seasoned Woman*, Gail Sheehy describes women between the ages of forty and ninety as "spicy," "seasoned," "marinated in life experience," and ". . . open to sex, love, dating, new dreams, exploring spirituality and revitalizing their marriages as never before." She calls this approach the Pursuit of a Passionate Life.[1] A woman that lives and feels this way is empowered, has hope, and gives aging a whole new meaning and direction.

Count your blessings. Think about the great things that your body does now. Yes, I said great things. Maybe it plays a mean game of golf? Walks your dogs? Does yoga? Snuggles your grandbabies? Holds your husband tight? Plays the piano? Plants daylilies? Bakes an astonishing apple cobbler? Make your own list. You'll find that, although your body has changed, it still does an incredible job for you and is a positive force in your life. Now that you're a bit older, a bit wiser, and have faced your own mortality, you can see your body from a broader perspective than you did twenty or thirty years ago. And because you now know you're not invincible, you won't take your body for granted anymore. In fact, heart disease can change your perspective on all of life's pleasures.

> *Enjoy and appreciate everything around you. It's funny how something like heart disease makes you appreciate your children, grandchildren, and the simple things in life even more.*
>
> —Margaret, Fresno, CA, age 36

---

1. Gail Sheehy, *Sex and the Seasoned Woman* (New York: Random House, 2006).

THE SCARS

I had to learn to accept my body and "love" my scars.
                                        —Mary, Cortlandt Manor, NY, age 54

Some women heart patients have scars from surgery that affect how they see themselves. Let's face it, they're not pretty. But you have nothing to be embarrassed or ashamed about. If that's how you feel, try to turn your thinking around. Give yourself time for your scars to heal. Eventually, they'll become a part of you just like your freckles or wrinkles. Try to think of each scar as a badge of courage—like battle scars—or as a symbol of your ability to survive. Many heart patients, ultimately, take pride in their scars because those scars prove that they're still here to enjoy and embrace life.

> *I was really bothered by this really ugly, large scar down the middle of my chest. It took about a year to adjust to the look of the scar and to feel okay about this new part of me. I have since had a scar revision and the look of the scar is much better. I have a much better, more positive outlook about my physical self. I'm no longer afraid to wear a V-neck sweater or a low-cut top. My whole body image has improved by huge leaps.*
>
> —Anna, Indianapolis, IN, age 48

In Anna's case, a scar revision was an important way to help her feel better, because it helped her self-image. If you're concerned about the physical appearance of your scar, your cardiologist can refer you to a surgeon who can help you. In some cases, the surgeon can actually remove wires and staples.

Sometimes, a scar revision is necessary to relieve discomfort. About a year after my bypass surgery, I had lost some weight and I could swear the staples were protruding through my skin. The discomfort was real but I wasn't sure if it was from the staples or something else. I ran into my cardiologist at a meeting and told her about it. Even then, I didn't fully trust my own judgment. Was this something I was imagining? We found a ladies room nearby and she took a look; then she felt the scar—and she too could feel the staples. "Go see your cardiac surgeon," she said. "Find out what he can do to help you." Sure enough, my surgeon was able to take most of the staples out without a problem and improve my scar a bit. Not incidentally, he told me protruding staples were a common problem. I'll tell you I wasn't thrilled about going under the knife *again* but he assured me that, this time, I wouldn't have to have that awful tube put down my throat and I could just have an intravenous (IV) sedation. Within about a month or two after the scar surgery, the difference in my chest discomfort was dramatic.

Another common problem with scars comes with sleeping discomfort. I have spoken to dozens of women who have had bypass or valve replacement surgery and the majority of them have a strange sensation when they sleep on their left side. One morning I woke up startled out of a sound sleep by an intense pain on the left side of my chest. The discomfort was near my scar, it made it hard to breathe and radiated across the left side of my chest. I knew I wasn't having a heart attack because the symptoms were different but it still was a very scary morning. I went right to my cardiologist, who found nothing wrong and reassured me that such aches are not uncommon. She did multiple tests to make sure there was nothing medically wrong.

Many women heart patients report these types of strange sensations, discomforts, and at times pain, especially on their left side. The pain is from scar tissue, nerve damage, and the fact that the pericardium of the heart was cut for the surgery, affecting the way the heart is held in the chest cavity.[2]

> *Simply cutting the sternum open or using an artery in the chest wall for a bypass procedure can result in chronic pain or discomfort. For many women, this discomfort can make it difficult to distinguish between a heart event and scar pain. If you're experiencing any kind of chronic pain or discomfort, it's important to address it with your doctor. Don't suffer in silence. Talk to your doctor about treatment options.*
>
> —Stacy C. Smith, MD, FACC

2. E. Eisenberg, Y. Pultorak, D. Pud, and Y. Bar-El, "Prevalence and Characteristics of Post Coronary Artery Bypass Graft Surgery Pain (PCP)," *Pain* 92 (1–2) (May 2001): 11–17.

Scars can cause discomfort—sometimes for many years. If you have a problem with the way your scar feels or looks, go to your cardiologist and see if he or she can help you, or refer you to someone who can. There's no reason to think of it as being "all in your head." It's better to be evaluated by your cardiologist than to worry or be afraid that something else is going on. In some instances—like the sleep discomfort on the left side—it may just be something you have to adjust to; you might have to find sleeping positions that are comfortable for you. But any time you experience ongoing discomfort, it's important to discuss your options with your doctor.

TAKING CARE OF YOURSELF

What can you do to lift yourself up? Make a conscious effort to take care of yourself. For starters, eat a heart-healthy diet. You'll feel better and look better. Get out of the house and do something special—just for you—on a regular basis. It can help boost your confidence and self-esteem. When you actively build confidence, you enhance your body image and begin to feel sexier, more desirable, and more attractive. Here are a few things that can jump-start your self-esteem:

- Go to an exercise or yoga class.
- Get your hair done.
- Get a makeover.
- Shop for a new outfit.
- Go out to lunch with some good friends.
- Surround yourself with those you care about.
- Spend time with the people who make you feel good about yourself—and avoid the people who don't.

REDUCING STRESS

Stress happens. You can't completely eliminate it from your life. You may not know it, but stress can either be positive or negative. If you get a new job, that's positive stress. If you lose your job, that's negative stress. Chronic stress is bad for your health. Ultimately, it's all about how you handle it. Here are a few things you can do to help reduce stress:

PAMPER YOURSELF

There is no need to go to India or anywhere else to find peace. You will find that deep place of silence right in your room, in your garden . . .
—Elisabeth Kübler-Ross

Oftentimes women are too busy with all their responsibilities to stop and smell the roses. Taking care of others at your own expense can be costly to your body image and self-esteem. Here are some ideas for indulging yourself:

- Take a bubble bath. Light candles, listen to soft music, and breathe deeply.
- Read a good book. And don't let anyone interrupt you.
- Do a crossword puzzle. And savor a nice cup of tea.
- Go sit in your garden and just enjoy the air, the sun, and the breeze.
- Take a walk in the park by yourself, with a dog, a friend, or your family. Use all of your senses while you're there.
- Get a pedicure or manicure. Or get your hair done.
- Have a massage, a facial, or some other delightful spa treatment.
- Buy yourself flowers.
- Sit by a fire.
- Take a nap (but not for more than sixty minutes).
- Go to the movies.
- Eat a piece of delicious dark chocolate.

- *Use proven stress-reduction techniques.* Yoga and meditation are widely accepted approaches to help reduce stress. There are books, videos, CDs, and classes in most communities that teach you how to integrate these techniques into your life. If you find that you're experiencing stress, you'll want to look into these options. For a quick fix, try the relaxation techniques on page 95. Of course, exercise is another proven stress reducer—and that's a must-do for every heart patient.
- *Clean up the messes in your life—literally and figuratively.* So often we choose avoidance as a way of dealing with our responsibilities,

relationships, and emotions. If a closet needs straightening, clean it out. Throw out all that unnecessary stuff you've been saving—and mend what needs fixing. Imagine how good you will feel when you're finished!

- *The same holds true for relationships.* If a relationship needs repairing, make the phone call and try to fix the problem. Try to let go and forgive. When you do, you'll not only free yourself, you'll also release the other person. Remember, no one is perfect. All of us make mistakes and hurt others either directly or indirectly. Take the bull by the horns and take active steps to resolve those conflicts. It might be a rough ride, but in the end everyone will be relieved and feel better. (Of course, there are some people with whom you won't be able to resolve your conflicts. See Chapter 7.)

- *Embrace your spirituality*—and I don't just mean your religion. Knowing that there's something greater than yourself can give you a sense of peace and anchor you in the moment. Spirituality is how you see yourself in the world and your place in it. You can feel spiritual just witnessing a sunset, a falling star, or a flower in bloom. Any time you feel a sense of awe, it can be a spiritual experience. Just let yourself take it all in!

- *Cultivate your sense of humor.* Laughter can help keep things in perspective, minimizing the importance of whatever it is that stresses you out. Find ways to bring laughter into your life every day. Read the comics. Rent a comedy. Look for the humor in situations, and try to cultivate relationships with people who make you laugh. Believe it or not, studies show that laughter is good for your heart! [3]

- *Try to find balance in your life.* A good motto to live by is: Too much of any one thing is not good for you. Or, as my grandmother used to say, everything in moderation. If you work too hard, play too hard, or do any one thing too much of the time, chances are it will take a toll on your sense of well-being. Try to set aside time in your busy day for yourself, to relax, rejuvenate,

---

3. "Laughter is good for your heart, according to new University of Maryland Medical Center Study," *University of Maryland Medical News*, November 15, 2000, http://www.umm.edu/news/releases/laughter.html.

rest, and exercise. Make taking care of yourself—and enjoying and appreciating life—a priority.

TEN WAYS TO REDUCE STRESS

1. Take a yoga class. You kill two birds with this stone. It will reduce your stress and enhance your body image.
2. Meditate. Take a class or use a how-to video, CD, or book to train yourself.
3. Take a nap, but try not to sleep for more than an hour or you'll wake up more tired than you were originally.
4. Exercise regularly (see Chapter 4).
5. Write in a journal. Brainstorm your feelings and get them on paper. Then problem-solve by making a list of things you can do to reduce your stress.
6. Vent to a trusted friend or clergy member.
7. Get psychotherapy to learn better techniques to manage your emotions, stress, and anger.
8. Join a support group (see Chapter 3 to find out how).
9. Listen to music in a quiet place where you can't be disturbed. You'll want to turn off all your phones and your computer, if it's nearby.
10. Make sure you get enough sleep every night. It's recommended you get about eight hours per night. If you're having trouble sleeping, speak to your doctor.

RELAXATION TECHNIQUES

Try these relaxation techniques that you can do anywhere:

- *Deep breathing.* Breathe in through your nose and out your mouth. Breathe slowly and deeply—for example, silently count to ten as you take in your first breath. You should feel your abdominal muscles move up and down when you breathe this way. Don't just use your upper chest. Pull the air all the way through your body. Breathe like this ten times and you will feel more relaxed.

PET THERAPY

You know the old saying, "Dogs are a man's best friend." Well, it's no joke. Studies show that pets can help to soothe people, improve mood, reduce blood pressure, and reduce stress. Of course, animal lovers and owners already know what the research is now confirming: Our furry friends provide us with unconditional love and affection, which in turn gives us social support and comfort. In addition, dogs give us a reason to go out and exercise, and keep us company in the process. So having pets is good for you, even though they're an added responsibility.

Sources: www.webmd.com/content/Article/115/111638.htm; http://stress.about.com/od/lowstresslifestyle/a/petandstress.htm; American Heart Association Scientific Sessions 2005, Dallas, Nov. 13–16, 2005: Kathie Cole, RN, University of California Medical Center in Los Angeles, Sidney Smith Jr., MD, American Heart Association spokesman, Professor of Medicine, University of North Carolina at Chapel Hill.

- *Total relaxation.* Close your eyes. Contract and relax the muscles in your body from your head to your toes. Visualize your muscles tensing and relaxing. Really think about telling each muscle group to relax—your legs, abdomen, chest, arms, and so forth—right down to your fingers and toes. Each time you contract a muscle group, hold it a few seconds, then release. This exercise will make you feel rejuvenated.
- *Visualization.* Close your eyes. Sit comfortably in a chair. Imagine yourself lying on a towel on the beach with the wind softly blowing and the sun shining warmly on your skin. Hear the ocean as it hits the beach. Feel the warm sand between your toes and your fingers. Visualize yourself there for just a few minutes. When you're finished, you will feel ready to face the world again.

THE SEXUAL SELF

A chicken and an egg are lying in bed. The chicken is smoking a cigarette with a satisfied smile on its face and the egg is frowning and looking out. The egg mutters to no one in particular, "I guess we answered the question."

—Author Unknown

Wouldn't it be great if understanding sex was really that easy? Body image and sex are intimately connected. The better you feel about your body, the more comfortable you are with sex. Women with heart disease are grappling not only with a new image of their bodies, they face a variety of fears and anxieties.

Some women heart patients are afraid they might die if they have intercourse or an orgasm. They're afraid they'll experience chest pain or some other pain during sex. Others fear that, with their scars or midlife body changes, they'll no longer excite their partner—or even that their bodies are, somehow, no longer physically capable of having sex. They think their sex life is over—that they're too old for such things. Sometimes women heart patients just feel unmotivated and too tired to be interested in sex. And they're too embarrassed to talk to their partner or their doctor about sex.

If you're experiencing some of these feelings, the problem can become magnified by the fact that your partner may have similar fears. Unfortunately, all the anxiety and discomfort your body has experienced can make sex seem foreign and strange. And given everything else that's going on in your life, it's all too easy to put sex on the back burner.

It's important to know that all these fears are normal and will fade over time. The good news is that having a heart event or being middle aged doesn't mean your sex life is over. Research has shown that nearly 40 percent of postmenopausal women with heart disease have active sex lives.[4] In fact, sex can be better than it's ever been for you and your partner. This may be a perfect opportunity to improve and rekindle the intimacy and romance in your relationship and your sex life.

You'll be able to gradually resume your full sex life—and I'll walk you through that process. But first let me allay your fears about dying or having another heart event during or after sex. According to the American Heart Association (AHA), there is no truth to the myth that you will have another heart attack or die suddenly if you resume having sex. The AHA recommends that heart patients resume sexual activity as soon as they feel ready.[5] In fact, one recent study showed that there's no more risk

---

4. I. B. Addis, C. C. Ireland, E. Vittinghoff, et al., "Sexual Activity and Function in Postmenopausal Women with Heart Disease," *Obstetrics & Gynecology* 106 (2005): 121–27.

5. Sexual Activity and Heart Disease and Stroke, AHA Recommendations, June 8, 2006, www.americanheart.org.

from sexual activity among people who have had heart events than among those with no history of heart disease.[6]

Your risk of having a heart event during or after sex is reduced further—whether or not you have heart disease—if you exercise for thirty minutes daily with moderate intensity or conditioning workouts, such as walking, swimming, biking, or dancing. Exercise also boosts your self-confidence, enhances your self-esteem, and makes you feel more desirable.

TALK TO YOUR DOCTOR FIRST

Every heart patient is different. We all have different medical conditions and concerns. And it's always wise to err on the side of safety. So always talk to your cardiologist first. If your cardiologist doesn't bring up the issue of sex with you, then you should bring it up. If you're uncomfortable or embarrassed talking to your doctor about sex, consider changing physicians. You should be able to talk with your cardiologist about all your worries and fears. In fact, it's critical. Be your own best health advocate and speak up. It's too important a topic to stay quiet and suffer in silence.

Just ask your cardiologist when it's okay to have sex again. Typically, your doctor will give you a time frame and a physical goal that you need to reach first before having sex—such as climbing a few flights of stairs without chest pain or having several uneventful weeks in your cardiac rehabilitation program. Your cardiologist can do tests in the office to reassure you that you are physically ready to have sex.

TAKE IT SLOW

I had my heart attack in February and it took me until April to try to have sex. I was terrified. While my husband and I were in the middle of having sex, I burst into tears and told him to stop. I was so afraid that I would have another heart attack. Since I didn't have a bypass, I had no problem with my body image. But sex terrified me. Even though I now know that sex will not cause me to have another heart attack, I feel different and changed. I will

---

6. J. Brody, "Heart Patients Need Not Fear Sex, Study Finds," *New York Times,* May 8, 1996.

never fully experience sex the same way I did before my heart at-
tack. No doctor has discussed this issue with me. I'm still strug-
gling with this.

—Rachel, Jamaica, NY, age 52

After a heart event, you may have to reconnect with your sexual self again before you can even think about being intimate with your partner. Remember, things have likely changed for you emotionally and physically since your event. It's important to know what pleases you sexually and that may mean self-exploration. Learn about your body; know what you like, when and where. You can build your confidence by masturbating and testing the waters with your own body before you involve a partner. Then, when you're ready, communicate those needs to your partner. If you learn to love your body, your partner will too and your anxiety will diminish.

In the beginning, I had a hard time looking at myself in the mir-
ror—with such deep, dark scars on me. Three years later, my scars
are beginning to fade. I've been intimate. I'm beginning to under-
stand that how I feel and see myself on the inside is so much more
important than what's going on with my body on the outside. I'm
single, never married, and am involved with someone now. But
it's hard to say where it'll lead. Children are probably not the
greatest idea for me. Intimacy is still difficult sometimes due to
the physical limitations from my bypass surgery. But it's nice to
know now that I have a man in my life who's sympathetic and ac-
cepting of me. I think underneath it all you need time, a spiritual
center, and a positive outlook and support to make it through and
to find your way back to feeling (and looking) like a beautiful, at-
tractive, sexy, and vibrant woman. And I'm still on my way!

—Sarah, West Hempstead, NY, age 29

Sex is not just about having intercourse. It's not just about physical sensations. It's much more complicated than that. For most women, getting in the mood has more to do with her frame of mind and her emotions than her sex organs. For many women, foreplay involves the way a partner lovingly and playfully interacts with her, touches and holds her in an embrace that says it all, and speaks to her with that soft and loving voice.

Your relationship outside the bedroom can have a real impact inside the bedroom. If your partner tries to make your life easier by helping around the house without being asked and thinking about your needs in general, that can be a real turn-on. It's amazing how women respond to their partners when their "honey-do" list is taken care of. It can help a woman relax and put her in the mood for lovemaking. It promotes emotional intimacy. And that emotional connection is just as important as the stimulation that comes with physical intimacy like kissing, touching, and caressing.

Give yourself time to heal physically and emotionally. Negative emotions can get in the way of your interest in sex. Most of these feelings and moods will subside over a three-month period after your heart event. But if you remain depressed for a longer period, you're likely to have less interest in sex, have sex less frequently and enjoy it less when you do.[7][8][9] There's no reason for you to have to suffer. Seek counseling as soon as possible. (See Chapter 3, Getting the Help you Need.)

> *Prior to my diagnosis of heart disease, I had been uninterested in sex. It was a struggle to get in the mood and the act itself just turned me off. This of course was frustrating to my husband and myself. I not only had a blocked artery but I was blocking feelings too. We had many, many personal things happening in our lives at the time; it was easy to dismiss sex. After my bypass, I was afraid to have sex because I was worried that if I got excited I could have another heart attack or something worse might happen. Emotionally I have made huge leaps about my fears, but this was done through the process of therapy. My self-image has improved and I have much more interest in having sex. I'm not afraid anymore and can have fun and enjoy myself in all facets of my life.*
>
> —Anna, Indianapolis, IN, age 48

It may be that intercourse, oral sex, or orgasm won't happen for many weeks. Take it slow. Just touching, cuddling, fondling, and kissing without

---

7. Sex and Heart Disease, www.stlukesonline.org/services/heart/images/sex.pdf.

8. Sex and Your Heart, 2002, www.justmove.org/fitnessnews/hfbodyframe
.cfm?Target=sexandheat.html.

9. Wayne Sotile, PhD, with Robin Cantor-Cooke, *Thriving with Heart Disease* (New York: Free Press, 2003).

the goal of having an orgasm may be a good place to start. Enjoy this low-key approach, embrace the newness, and have fun. You may have to learn something new to please your partner or yourself. Make sure you are totally comfortable and ready before you move on to other forms of sexual contact.

There's no need for you or your partner to have marathon sex out of the gate. Set the mood before you begin. Make sure there's peace and quiet, maybe soft music playing. Prop up the pillows, make adjustments for comfort. Make sure you are well rested and aren't stressed. Just like jumping in a pool after you eat, it's better to wait one to three hours after you eat before having sex. If you're sexually active, be especially careful to take your medication as directed by your physician. For example, some women find that, if they haven't taken their medication yet and they engage in sexual activity—particularly right before bed or first thing in the morning—they experience symptoms. That can be scary (see page 102, How to Tell If It's an Emergency).

You may have other physical issues you need to address. For example, women in midlife frequently have difficulties with vaginal lubrication, which makes intercourse uncomfortable or painful. There are all sorts of products out there for this common problem. An Ob/Gyn doctor, Ob/Gyn nurse practitioner, or a sexoligist can help you wade through the many solutions that exist.

As with so many other aspects of your life with heart disease, sexual positions and activities may have to change too. Some sexual activities require more physical energy than others. An Ob/Gyn doctor, Ob/Gyn nurse practitioner, or a sexoligist can give you recommendations for sexual positions and alternatives that might make you more comfortable, stress your body less, and build your confidence. It's possible that, for a while, you and your partner will want to please each other through mutual masturbation or oral sex, which is less physically taxing on the body than intercourse. Anal sex is not recommended because it's been shown to affect heart rhythms and blood pressure.[10] [11]

Remember, it's normal for you and your partner to feel vulnerable and scared after your heart event, so be patient with each other. Try to be a source of mutual comfort and tenderness for one another. Reassure each other, experiment, laugh, play, and enjoy the intimacy.

> *The first time I made love to my husband following my bypass surgery was scary. To me it was almost like the first time I had*

sex. I could not relax. I wondered if my chest would hurt. I wanted to make my husband feel comfortable, so I tried to act normal. I remember thinking you have to breathe—DO NOT HOLD YOUR BREATH! I had finished cardiac rehab, so I was not concerned that I would have another heart attack. Since I was only forty-five and newly married, I wanted to reassure my husband that everything would be the way it was before. Now I realize that I was the one who needed reassurance. He wasn't worried a bit. Men!

—Ashley, Phoenix, AZ, age 48

Of course communication is critical to having a healthy and happy sex life. If you communicate your needs, wants, and feelings with each other, it's likely that you'll improve your emotional intimacy, reduce your stress, and improve your sex life. No matter how long you've been with your partner, don't assume anything. Make an effort to communicate. Check things out and ask questions. Talk to each other. And if you need it, get counseling.

The combination of aging and heart disease can have a dramatic impact on a woman's body, image, self-esteem, and inner peace. Through

HOW TO TELL IF IT'S AN EMERGENCY

When you start making love, you will experience the normal body changes associated with sex—increased heart rate, heavier breathing, and flushed skin. But be aware of and alert to the following symptoms:

- Significant shortness of breath.
- Pressure, pain, or discomfort in your chest, neck, jaw, arm, or stomach.
- Irregular or very rapid heartbeats.

Use common sense. If these symptoms happen, stop, rest, and see if the symptoms subside. If they do not subside, take your emergency medications as prescribed. If the pain continues for more than fifteen minutes, call 911 and go directly to the emergency room. Whether your symptoms subside or not, be sure to notify your doctor about your experience.

actively pursuing ways to reduce your stress and fears and by reconstructing your sense of self as a vibrant, passionate, and attractive woman, you'll have a more fulfilling sex life, an improved sense of yourself, and a more intimate relationship with those you love.

> *You gain strength, courage, and confidence by every experience in which you really stop to look fear in the face. You must do the thing which you think you cannot do.*
>
> —Eleanor Roosevelt

WHEN TO SEEK SUPPORT

Any of the following can interfere with your sex life:

- *Medications.* Blood pressure or fluid pills, tranquilizers, antidepressants, and some other cardiac medications. Check with your doctor regarding potential side effects.
- *Psychological issues.* Depression, fear, sadness, sleep difficulties, body weight changes, fatigue, change in eating habits, lack of interest, inability to relax, bad timing, and other life stressors can all affect your interest in resuming sex. Chapter 2 addresses some of these issues in detail.
- *Previous relationship issues.* A history of sexual problems, marital conflicts, legal concerns, financial problems, or family troubles.

If any of these issues are affecting your interest in or your ability to resume sex, seek help as soon as possible. Talk to your partner and communicate your feelings, try to figure out what the problems are and try to discuss possible solutions. If this doesn't help, get counseling as soon as possible before the problems become more difficult to resolve. (See Chapter 3 for guidance.) Talk to your doctor about the effects of your medications. No matter what, do not stop your medications before you speak to your doctor or health-care provider.[12] [13] [14]

---

12. Sex and Heart Disease.

13. Sex and Your Heart, 2002.

14. Sotile and Cantor-Cooke, *Thriving with Heart Disease.*

WHAT SEX CAN DO FOR YOU

- Builds your confidence and self-esteem.
- Is a life-affirming act—a reminder that you are still vibrant and alive.
- Reinforces the fundamental belief that your body can still function well and that you can feel good despite heart disease.
- Helps you to regain a sense of normalcy and wholeness.
- Relieves headaches and improves your mood (thanks to those endorphins or neurohormones.)
- Improves your appearance. When you release estrogen after making love it makes your hair shine and your skin smooth.
- Gives you a bit of a workout. Sex burns calories, and stretches and tones your body.
- Helps you relax. It's a great, natural tranquilizer.

THE NEXT STEP

Your sex life isn't the only thing at home that feels different. Your family probably imagined everything would go back to normal once you physically recovered from your heart event. But it didn't. How do you help them change their expectations? How can you communicate effectively—but differently? It may involve redefining roles within the family. The next chapter will explain how and address some of the tougher issues associated with your family life after a heart event.

chapter six

COPING WITH CHANGE

Your Family

You don't choose your family. They are God's
gift to you, as you are to them.
—Desmond Tutu

My youngest son, Jon, is fourteen. One day I told him I was working on this chapter and I was struggling with how to explain how complex families are, that they function as a system based on rules, roles, traditions, history, and genes—not to mention all those personalities. I was trying to imagine how to explain it without getting too complicated and too far afield. And he said, "Don't worry, Mom. It's simple. Families are like most of nature: everything is interrelated and interconnected. One thing influences the next; that's life." As my jaw dropped, I realized how right he was about families.

So, courtesy of my son Jon, I invite you to think of your family as a rain forest. Look at it this way: If one tree is diseased or is cut down, it affects all the birds and plants and animals—the flora and fauna—that surround that tree. That ecosystem will eventually adapt without the tree. It will reestablish itself and regain its balance, but it will take time. That's pretty much the way families operate. If one person gets sick, it affects every member of the family. And like an ecosystem that experiences a disruption, a family will try to regain its balance. But that, too, takes time.

Families have as many configurations as constellations in the sky—and how different families handle an illness and try to find a balance can be just as varied. Families are fluid—shifting and changing to adapt to life's ups and downs. When an illness strikes, some families will rise to the occasion, stronger in the face of it. Others will struggle and seem to fall apart. Every family will react a bit differently. But you can count on one thing: At first, a heart event will put any family into a crisis mode, creating chaos and turmoil. That couldn't be more normal.

Once you go home from the hospital, you can expect everything to be out of sync for a while. For one thing, your illness has changed how your family sees you—and what they expect of you. And your expectations of them have changed as well. You may treat each other differently or talk to each other differently. The roles of the various family members may shift. Suddenly an older child may take on more responsibility. A younger one may become insecure and clingy. A grandparent may move in for a while. A husband—or even an ex-husband—may become more of a caregiver. Relatives—even members of your immediate family—may become over-bearing and intrusive. All kinds of roles, patterns, routines, behaviors, and, ultimately, relationships may change.

For some women and their families, these changes will be temporary. For others, they'll be significant and lasting. But every family will experi-ence some degree of change. So get ready. Once you simply accept the fact that there are changes afoot, you can begin to work together as a family to get through it in a positive way.

ONE DAY AT A TIME

My family had a terrible time at first. They treated me like a little fragile glass slipper on a satin pillow. That drove me insane. And I'll never forget the first week home from the hospital; everyone took turns bringing our dinner. We had baked chicken every single night.
—Tasha, Hot Springs, AR, age 40

Your family generally takes over during your first weeks at home. In all likelihood, they're communicating with one another to make sure you're being taken care of. Maybe your mother or sister has come to town to help. Or your husband's taken a week off from work. For a while, friends and neighbors may be feeding the family, dropping off casseroles, and, of course, all that chicken. You may find yourself at the center of a kind of caregiving frenzy. All this activity gives your family a sense of control over a difficult situation.

During those first weeks, it's important to set realistic expectations for your household. What's important? Two things. First, you want your kids' lives to be as normal as possible. That might mean making sure they get to school and activities, that there's food on the table, and the laundry's done. Second, anything that relates to your immediate recovery is a top priority—getting to all your doctor's appointments, getting the rest you need, and following your doctor's orders, whatever they may be. Everything else becomes secondary.

If your family has a complex and busy schedule, you may find yourself giving instructions, date book in hand: "Cancel Adam's dentist appointment on Tuesday. But be sure he gets to soccer on Friday." There are probably things you won't be able to do for a while: drive your car, pick up grocery bags, lift the laundry basket. At that point, you need a great deal of help and support.

Gradually, though, things will change. Your doctor may tell you that you can drive. He'll probably encourage you to increase your level of activity every day. Maybe you'll start cardiac rehab. Maybe you'll begin doing a few things around the house. But as time passes you'll be able to do more.

As this process unfolds, you and your family will have to adapt and change—again and again and again. Here are some guidelines to help you through this process, so your family can regain its footing.

Talk Talk Talk

At first I was treated like a china doll and not allowed to breathe for my family's fear that I'd keel over. We have become closer and more open with one another. We're all more aware of the disease and are working on being healthier. We talk, talk, talk, and I've had to learn when to just listen, and when to just touch. They've learned not to be so protective of me. And as time goes by they're

*not as jumpy as they were at first. I'm not as fragile in their
minds anymore.*

—Anna, Indianapolis, IN, age 48

With all of the stress that you and your family have been through, one of
the most important things you can do is to communicate your needs to
your family. Think of this as an opportunity to improve your relationships
and communication skills. If you're a woman who's always done just about
everything for your family and you now have to give up some of your previous roles, it's imperative that you find a calm and collected way to talk to
your family about these changes. If you wait and expect them to read your
mind, you'll feel let down, disappointed that they don't know things have
to change—and that you can't and shouldn't do it all anymore.

Don't expect your family to know that changes need to be made for
your health and to reduce your stress.

Tell them what you can and can't do.   Your family won't know, from day to
day, how you're feeling, and what you can and can't do. So it's very important to talk to them. They'll see you begin to get up and around. For
example, at first, your family may have to go with you to the grocery
store. Then, at some point, you can go yourself. They'll probably worry
about you. They won't want you to do too much, to overstress yourself.
Of course, that's because they love you. It's your responsibility to let them
know what you're capable of doing. You might just say: "Don't worry. I
can handle the grocery shopping now. The doctor says it's okay." So keep
in mind: It's your responsibility to educate and communicate what you're
able to do physically.

Conversely, if you need help and there's something you can't do, it's
important to let them know. And to ask for help. Don't expect them to
read your mind or anticipate all your needs. Sometimes that just means
getting someone's help to unload the groceries ("Honey, I'm not supposed to lift heavy packages, so I'll need your help.") Sometimes that applies to the emotional realm as well.

Talk to them about how to communicate more effectively with one another.
It's important for heart patients to limit the amount of stress they're under. That means you have to limit arguments and fighting. If your kids are

fighting, you need to talk to them. Tell them it's not good for them and it's not good for you. The family needs to function as a team. You might say: "I'm not trying to scare you, but these kinds of fights are not good for my heart. It's unhealthy for you, too. We need to do better. We have to change how we relate to one another."

It's important for the entire family to find ways to resolve conflict—ways that work for everyone. Create outlets to resolve conflicts. Some approaches you might consider include family conferences to talk through the issues; time-outs where people go to separate areas of the house for a cooling-off period. Individuals may want to try going for a walk, writing in a journal or drawing or painting to calm down in the wake of a conflict. Making a conscious effort to reduce conflict can dramatically improve relationships.

The same holds true for marriages. If you and your partner tend to scream and yell, you need to work together to change that pattern. If those conflicts represent more than a communication style, you need to address the underlying problem. At least one study has shown that people who are highly satisfied in their marriages are less likely to develop metabolic syndrome, which is linked to cardiovascular disease.[1] Conversely, research tells us that marital stress puts women heart patients at risk for a recurrence.[2] Knowing that marital satisfaction impacts on your heart health gives you important information. If you are unhappy and dissatisfied in your marriage, don't ignore it. Seek counseling as soon as possible. (See Chapter 3 for guidance on finding help.)

Tell them that you're still available to them. Your family may be feeling all kinds of worries and stresses—feelings they may not want to share with you for fear that it might make your heart problems worse. Your family needs to know that they're still at the top of your priority list, and that if they've got any questions or concerns about anything, you're still there for them.

---

1. W. M. Troxel, K. A. Matthews, L. C. Gallo, et al., "Marital Quality and Occurrence of the Metabolic Syndrome in Women," *Archives of Internal Medicine* 165 (2005): 1022–27.

2. K. Orth-Gomer, S. P. Wamala, M. Horsten, K. Schenck-Gustafsson, N. Schneiderman, and M. A. Mittleman, "Marital Stress Worsens Prognosis in Women with Coronary Heart Disease: The Stockholm Female Coronary Risk Study," *JAMA-Journal of the American Medical Association* 284 (2000): 3008–14.

Don't expect perfection. A word of caution: Encouraging communication by being honest and open doesn't mean you won't get flack from your family, or have conflicts, bouts of guilt, anger, or resentment. We're all only human. The point is: Try to be conscious of everyone's feelings and the fact that you're all under stress.

> *As a Native American woman, my family is the center. Some-times our balance is off but mostly we are there for each other. We may not always agree how I handle my illnesses at times. My daughters have very different personalities but they are kind-hearted and thoughtful women. But they do worry about me and sometimes are rough on me. I let them know that I'm still here for them no matter what. We are there for each other to work it out together. As we say in our culture, "it's all in a good way, from a good place, and from a good heart."*
>
> —Wanda, Menifee, CA, age 61

EDUCATE YOUR FAMILY ABOUT HEART DISEASE

> *Men need to be equipped through education to become better lis-teners to their wife's utterances of symptoms, whether vague or clearly stated. They can be terrific advocates and supporters, help-ing to make sure that their loved one is receiving the proper diag-nosis and treatment, if they were only properly informed!*
>
> —Mary's husband Bill, Mesa, AZ, age 69

One way to help family members understand your needs is by giving them articles and books to read on the subject of women and heart dis-ease. Those educational tools can get your family up to speed on potential issues and address their concerns. Send them to www.womenheart.org, where they can find answers to their questions and order books and edu-cational materials, or to one of these other Web sites for information and ma-terials: www.hearttruth.gov, www.4woman.gov, www.americanheart.org, or www.hearthealthywomen.org.

> *My pride and joy are my grandchildren—five boys and a girl. They all know about my illnesses. We just want them to live their*

lives. It's better that way. But my daughters have made great strides by changing their families' lifestyle choices, since they've become aware of our family history and the dangers. It's good that they know and are doing something about it.

—Wanda, Menifee, CA, age 61

BE AS LOVING AND REASSURING AS YOU CAN BE

Don't underestimate the power of kindness and affection. I'll never forget that February day five years ago when I came home from the hospital. It was snowing in Memphis—yes, I said snowing in Memphis! No one had expected me to go home so soon, but I was determined. Of course, my doctor told me that I had to show him I could walk the halls before he would discharge me. I walked and walked—and he let me go home even though I still had drainage tubes in from my bypass surgery. It turned out to be a day of fabulous coincidences. I hadn't seen my kids in six days and there was nothing I wanted more than to be with them. And because of

---

HOW TO ASK YOUR FAMILY TO HELP

Remember: Use "I" messages instead of "you" messages. This sends a signal that you're respectful of the listener and taking responsibility for your feelings and behavior. "I" messages diffuse intense situations and emotions. For instance, in talking to your kids you could say, "I feel tired and need your help for the next few months, until I feel better. Jon, I need you to help me by taking out the trash every week. Nathaniel, if you fill the dishwasher after dinner that would give me time to sit down and relax. Ben, if you could stop by the grocery store once a week to bring a few items home that would be a great help to me. I know you're not used to me asking you to do these types of things but now I need your help, so I can get better and things will get done. We all need to work together. I love you guys!" If they balk, be patient, kind, and acknowledge their feelings, but stick to the plan and don't buckle under the pressure. They can handle what you're asking them to do—you just have to make it happen.

MEN VERSUS WOMEN: GENDER STUDIES

Studies provide plenty of evidence that it's important for women to be assertive and ask for help with household chores. Keep in mind that men and women think and communicate differently. If you want more help from your husband or partner, you have to be direct—and ask for it. Here are a few examples of what research tells us:

- In the weeks following a wife's heart attack, husbands did more chores than before—but wives still did as much as their husbands.[3]
- Women had a tendency to underplay their illness—they didn't want to bother their family with their health problems.[4]
- In general, male cardiac patients report more support from their spouses than women report.[5]
- Along the same lines, women received less information about the disease and rehabilitation than men received.[6]
- And women were more likely to experience a lack of belief in their heart problems from caregivers.[7]

What should you do? "Don't try to do too much, be sure to ask for help, and don't let other people underestimate your health concerns," says Dr. Shoshana Shiloh, PhD, Associate Professor of Psychology at Tel Aviv University. "Instead, use your illness and recovery as an opportunity for strengthening ties with the important people in your life—appreciate how much they care about you. Teach yourself to accept help from others without feeling guilty; and remind yourself that you'd be there if they needed your help."

---

3. Rose et al., "Comparison of Adjustment."

4. Ibid.

5. M. L. Kristofferzon, R. Lofmark, and M. Carlsson, "Myocardial Infarction: Gender Differences in Coping and Social Support," *Journal of Advanced Nursing* 44 (2003): 360–74.

6. Ibid.

7. Ibid.

the snow, school had been cancelled. None of us were supposed to be home, but that's where we all ended up.

I, of course, went straight to bed. But my kids came in one by one, asking me questions, showering me with hugs and kisses, and more questions. They kept coming in, climbing in bed with me, saying a few words, and asking a few questions. What are those tubes? When will you be able to get out of bed? Are you okay? My older son asked me how I felt. My youngest wanted to know if he'd miss soccer in the weeks ahead. And many of their questions reflected a general concern about when life was going to get back to normal. And if it was ever going to be normal again!

They'd ask a few questions and then they'd leave to go outside and play in the snow. They seemed to need to check in with me like this throughout the day; to touch me, to talk to me, to see that I was there and to feel reassured that I was okay—that Mommy was alive and really home.

I was exhausted and in some pain, but at the same time, I was incredibly moved by their visits. That made it one of the best days of my life. Their affection and concern made me feel better. And by reassuring them and empathizing with their concerns, I helped them feel better. And all those hugs and kisses were worth their weight in gold.

RECOGNIZE THAT YOUR FAMILY IS SCARED

My family has to know where I am at all times. If they can't reach me by phone they immediately think the worst has happened to me. They need their own support group to help them deal with living with a loved one who has heart disease.

—Rachel, Jamaica, NY, age 52

Fear and anxiety are a family's natural reactions to a heart event. I talked about the importance of empathy in Chapter 1. You can't have too much empathy. You need to try to empathize with your family members no matter how difficult that seems. Try to see things from their perspective. They will have intense emotional reactions to your heart event, and will need plenty of information and reassurance to begin to stop worrying about you and your health. It may seem odd for me to be asking you to take care of your family emotionally when you're the patient. But, as a woman, it's probably your natural tendency, and in the end it should help everyone adjust to all of the changes with a greater sense of security and less stress. Over time, your family's fear and anxiety should recede. Watching you get better is the best reassurance you can offer your family.

LET GO OF THE SUPERWOMAN THING

For a lot of women, it's particularly difficult to give up the role of super-woman. It takes time to learn to set realistic expectations for yourself—and for others. For starters, you'll likely have to make some changes in how you handle your household responsibilities. Put simply, you need to lower your expectations of what you can do. You're probably going to have to let other people help, and that means taking off some of the many hats you've always worn. So life will be a bit different. You might not be able to work, pay the bills, drive carpools, do all of the grocery shopping, cook all the meals, run the errands, take care of the yard work, volunteer, and love and nurture your family around the clock. I can already feel your anxiety level rising. Really. I hear the grunts and sighs from here. It may seem un-natural not to do all the things you're used to doing and it may be hard to let go of some of these tasks, but, in truth, you may have no choice.

Letting other people help also means giving up some control—and that may be the hardest part of all for some women. In order to give up

---

MAKE A JOB CHART

Spread the work out among your family members. Create a chart that tells everybody who will do what. Tell them why. Explain that you need more rest and you simply can't do as much right now—that it's important for your health and well-being. So you need their help. You may hear moans and complaints at first. But tell them how much you appreciate it. And that you know it's going to be hard for a while. But stick to your guns and get the help you need and deserve—it will be a teaching and growing experience for your family.

And it'll serve another purpose: It will make your kids more indepen-dent, responsible, and thoughtful about what it takes to run a family. Just re-member things might not get done exactly the way you would do them. That's when you take a deep breath, let go and move on.

control, you have to recognize that other people aren't going to do things exactly the way you do them. Whether your partner's cooking dinner or your daughter's mowing the lawn or your son's folding laundry or your mother-in-law is doing the grocery shopping, they're not necessarily going to do it your way. It's not necessarily going to be "perfect." That's something a lot of women have difficulty accepting. But letting others help you means letting go of preconceived notions of how something has to be done. Let them load the dishwasher from the left, fold the T-shirts their own way, and buy a different brand of dishwashing liquid. In the scheme of things, it's just not that important.

If guilt rears its ugly head, just realize that guilt is simply a warning signal telling you that things are changing. That's okay. That's the goal. Remind yourself that these changes are in everyone's best interest.

SET CLEAR BOUNDARIES

My first day at home, I wanted nothing more than to be surrounded by my children. But when you're sick, it's not unusual to find yourself surrounded by relatives who really aren't being helpful or who overstay their welcome. You're a captive audience and you need your rest. It's important that you set clear boundaries and expectations with your family—and that means all of your relatives. Here are a few examples of common boundary issues. A relative calls every two hours to check on you. That's intrusive and disrupts your ability to rest. Tell her, in the nicest way possible, to please limit her phone calls. Be specific. For example: "It's okay if you call every other day." Choose a time frame that works for you. Or say Aunt Ellen brings her friends over to visit without calling first. That's inappropriate and insensitive. Ask them to come back another time—but tell them to call first, because you might be resting or unavailable.

Sometimes relatives simply stay too long or ask too many inappropriate questions: Do you know when things are going to get back to normal? How is this going to affect your children? What does the doctor tell you—are you going to get better soon? Worse still, they offer advice that inflicts guilt or feels judgmental, like: "Why don't you stop working and just stay home with the kids?" Or "Maybe you shouldn't jog in the future." None of this is helpful. In fact, it makes you feel angry. What do you say? Tell them that you prefer that they not give you advice. Or say: "I know you care about me. But right now your advice isn't helping me."

Don't let any relative pressure you into saying more about yourself than you are comfortable sharing. Just tell them where you stand by saying, "Aunt Madge, I really don't feel comfortable sharing that with you. There are some things I only share with my husband and that's one of those things." She may end up giving you a "deer in the headlights" look but that's okay, you got her off your back for a moment. With relatives like Aunt Madge, you might have to rinse and repeat the same message multiple times for her to get the point. That's okay—you're entitled to keep your boundaries where you need them to be.

Recognize That Not Everyone Will Be Helpful

> *My siblings and I were in the mourning process of losing my mother six months before my heart attack. My sister's reaction in the ER when it didn't look like I was going to make it was, "No, Mom, you can't take her with you. We need her." I was always the "go-to" person for my siblings. That's had to change. They haven't changed but I have. They really don't know how to help me. It's hard on all of us.*
>
> —Ashley, Phoenix, AZ, age 48

Some people are natural-born caregivers. When I was recuperating, my sister-in-law came to visit from out of town. She sat with me and took care of me, and seemed to know exactly what to do. She made my lunch. She brought me a book about yoga. She and I would go for nice, quiet walks. Not everyone has that natural caregiving ability. Some people are awkward, even intimidated by illness. Others simply aren't very good at being helpful. They're the relatives who sit at the Thanksgiving table and let everyone else wait on them. Or they take a nap before dinner, while everyone else is working frantically to get things ready. You don't want these people around when you're not up to snuff.

How do you handle it? You—and your spouse or partner—can decide who should come to visit with you or help and who shouldn't. Then you let those relatives know—in a kind but clear way—that you've got enough help for now. Tell them that they can come visit when life is less

TEN SUCCESSFUL STRATEGIES FOR CONFLICT RESOLUTION

1. Take time away from the conflict to get perspective.
2. Get some advice from a trusted friend, family member, clergy, or therapist.
3. Most conflicts recur. Ask yourself if you need to deal with this conflict now or wait until it happens again. Or think about ways to avoid the same conflict in the future.
4. If you decide to address the conflict through a discussion, do it in person, if you can. Otherwise, talk on the phone. Never use e-mail to resolve a conflict—it leaves too much room for miscommunication.
5. Start the discussion on a positive note, such as, "It will make our relationship so much nicer if we can get through this," or "This issue keeps coming up again and again. It seems like things will be a lot calmer around here if we work it out."
6. Meet in a neutral and comfortable environment with few distractions.
7. Try to be as relaxed as possible and keep your demeanor calm.
8. Actively listen. Don't interrupt, and avoid blaming by using those "I" messages. And try to replay the other person's comments back to them. For instance, you can say, "Okay, just to help me understand, you're saying . . . ." or "Are you saying . . . let me make sure I'm hearing you correctly . . ." It shows that you're listening and understanding, which enhances communication and helps diffuse the tension.
9. Recognize that you may not end up agreeing with one another; but you might achieve a mutual understanding of the problem. It's always okay to agree to disagree.
10. If you're engaged in a discussion that isn't getting anywhere. Step away and give yourself more time to think about it. Say: "Let me give this some more thought, and we'll get back together and work this out."

difficult. You need and deserve to protect yourself from any unnecessary stress or discomfort.

THERE ARE POWERFUL STRESSORS AT WORK

> *One of the hardest things I have trouble getting a grip on is how heart disease has affected my family. When they treat me as if I'm fragile I get upset with them because I want to be "normal." When they dump things on me, I sometimes start feeling like "poor me"—don't they realize that I can't be Super Mom anymore?*
>
> *So even eight years after my first heart attack, we're still working things out.*
>
> —Ellen, Beverly Hills, MI, age 53

As I mentioned earlier, women are often the glue that holds their family together, the anchor or backbone that keeps things steady. Your family has an image of you and expectations of you. After all, you're the one that always took care of everything and everybody. And then you had a heart event, and those expectations and perceptions were disrupted and shifted. Not only are you not as available to take care of things as you once were, but also they're afraid they might lose you.

> *My husband of 22 years was standing in the ER beside me when I went into cardiac arrest. He witnessed them calling "Code Blue" and just as they were preparing the paddles to shock me, someone realized he was there and literally had to drag him out. I still have problems with the fact that he witnessed that.*
>
> —Tasha, Hot Springs, AR, age 40

We talked about loss and the grieving process in Chapter 2. You'll recall responses to loss run the gamut from denial and anger to sadness and guilt. Add the fear and anxiety that comes with having a heart patient in the family, and you've got a smorgasbord of emotional reactions. Then you add more stressors. As you begin to take care of yourself differently and change your priorities, your family members may find it difficult. They may feel neglected or even abandoned. They may balk at the changes in the family diet, or the fact that they have to take on new responsibilities, or the fact that you're taking a walk in the evening while they're doing the dishes.

All these reactions are perfectly natural. The entire family system feels loss when there is a change in roles, rules, and the expectations of the family. Acknowledging this loss to one another is very helpful in calming the turbulent waters during periods of change—and an important first step toward helping everyone adapt.

It's also important to make a conscious effort to address family issues. Say you notice an increase in angry remarks, or someone in your family just isn't acting like themself—maybe they're withdrawn or hostile or isolated from everyone else. If you start to feel that something's wrong, you'll want to address it right away. If it's an issue involving you and your husband, maybe the two of you can just go out to dinner and talk. If it involves the kids as well, you might want to have a family meeting. Go for a walk with everyone and clear the air. Maybe the problem is unrelated to you, but because you're not feeling well they're not telling you what's going on. They want to protect you. Or they may be feeling all kinds of worries and stresses—feelings they may not want to share with you for fear that it might make your heart problems worse. When problems arise, families have to make a conscious effort to get back to normal. Again, ongoing communication is central to that process.

When Denial Rears Its Head

Sometimes members of your family can be in denial, particularly your adult children or siblings. If they don't come over to visit, if they stay away or if they don't communicate, they may be in denial. They're just too afraid to talk about it. They may not want to deal with it because of their concern for you. Or they may not want to deal with it because they don't want to face the fact that they could have this same problem later in life.

> One obstacle I faced was dealing with my family. My sisters ignored my request for them to be tested for heart disease. One year later, my older sister ended up in a coma due to congestive heart failure. She was blessed in that she survived and her heart is functioning better now. Three months after my older sister's heart problem, my middle sister ended up with cardiomyopathy and she

*was told that she didn't have a great chance to survive beyond a
year. Both sisters are doing okay but if they had listened to me
maybe all of these incidents could have been prevented.*

—Lyn, Clearwater, FL, age 58

These situations can be frustrating. Recognizing that heart disease has
a family connection, you want to protect your family and make sure they
don't get sick. But they don't always listen. There's no point in getting angry with them or trying to force them to do something about their health.
It's not your responsibility. When it comes to concerns about their health,
you can offer advice and make suggestions. But how they want to handle
it is their choice. Beyond that, it's important to know that, if someone

---

HOW DO YOU JUDGE WHETHER IT'S AN UNHEALTHY SITUATION?

You'll want to make some changes, talk it out, or seek outside help if you
see any of the following warning signs.

- Kids become overinvolved or hypervigilant—watching over you or
  checking on you constantly.
- Family members are snapping at one another or saying mean things to
  each other most of the time.
- Someone seems depressed. Signs include withdrawing from everyone, and not wanting to get out of bed or to see friends. (See Chapter 2, page 34, for detailed symptoms of depression.)
- Signs of stress in younger children include bedwetting, inappropriate
  aggressive behavior, troubled sleep, or tantrums.
- For preteens and teenagers, stress can be expressed in acting-out behaviors, moodiness, or lower grades. They isolate themselves, stay
  away from their friends, or change their personal habits, such as their
  hygiene.
- If you just feel as if the family situation is out of control or someone in
  your family seems terribly stressed and unhappy, don't ignore it. Seek
  outside help if you need it. (See Chapter 3 for guidance on how to
  find outside help.)

doesn't come to see you or doesn't call, it may have more to do with them than with you.

BEWARE OF CAREGIVER BURNOUT

My husband, a reticent man by nature, has said relatively little about what he saw and felt as he witnessed my heart attack, which occurred in the ER, and when he saw me after emergency bypass surgery. But it's clear to me that he's suffered a great deal and that this experience has placed him under constant stress. Initially he treated me like an invalid. As my strength grew and my body healed, I began chafing under his excessive watchfulness. Slowly I convinced him that he had to let me resume my activities; that I could not heal nor could he, if I did not return to a more normal life. In many ways his life and mine have been fundamentally altered by his inability to relax with regard to my well-being.

—Mary, Cortlandt Manor, NY, age 54

Mary's experience with her husband is not an uncommon one. As I've mentioned before, the people who love you often experience deep fears and feelings of loss that are not unlike your own. That sense that things are spinning out of control is a feeling you probably share with your caregiver. Plus your caregiver has taken on the burden of a lot of new responsibilities—including things that he or she may never have done before. Sometimes a caregiver takes on too much and doesn't realize that they're setting themselves up for health or mental health problems. They can become overly burdened and forget to take care of themselves. The end result can be caregiver burnout.

My husband has been great. But there are days where I can tell that the whole thing seems to weigh heavily on him and the frustration he has knowing there is nothing he can do to fix this situation.

—Margaret, Fresno, CA, age 36

Think of all the ways your family's life has changed. You may not be able to do a lot of the things you could do before. And it's not just the household chores. You may have less energy and need more rest. You might even need help with the basics of personal care—getting dressed or bathing. Maybe you can't work anymore or pay the bills, and there are financial stresses. (See Chapter 8 for more on this issue.)

Your social life has surely changed—if only temporarily. Maybe you did a lot of entertaining before your heart event, or played mixed doubles every week with your husband. Maybe you went out to a pancake supper every Friday night with your sister. Or you and your boyfriend used to enjoy an evening at the ball game, eating hot dogs and drinking beer. Now your husband or your sister or your boyfriend has become your caregiver. And you can't do a lot of these things anymore.

> *I was really scared that I might mess up and let my wife die from a lack of knowing what to do. The stress was huge.*
> —Tina's husband Billy, Vaughn, MS, age 62

These changes and demands can put a strain on the relationship and on your entire family system. One study showed that a caregiving spouse can experience a higher level of anxiety and depression, and can feel less in control than the patient does—and that this can impact the patient's emotional and social well-being. In fact, a patient's social and emotional adjustment is significantly worse when the spouse is more anxious and depressed than the patient.[8]

Caregivers are grappling with all kinds of issues—the increased responsibilities; the feelings of loss and sadness; the frustration and sense that things are outside of their control; feelings of guilt that they're not doing more; and even a sense of an impending great loss. The fear of the unknown lingers. And they're worried about themselves—what will they do if they lose you? How long will the illness go on? How will it all affect them? They don't know what to expect from one day to the next. It can be very painful and difficult. And, not surprisingly, it can lead to burnout.

What can be done to prevent caregiver burnout?   There's nothing like a tender word or touch to diminish stress and anxiety. When my own mother was sick some years ago, I found solace in the depth of our mutual affec-

---

8. D. K. Moser and K. Dracup, "Role of Spousal Anxiety and Depression in Patients' Psychosocial Recovery after a Cardiac Event," *Psychosomatic Medicine* 66 (2004): 527–32.

tion. I could feel her loving me and nurturing me even when she wasn't feeling well. I felt it in her touch and in the way she looked at me. I knew I could make her feel better by holding her hand, or whispering a joke or something soothing in her ear. When two people love each other and knew each other well, the caregiving relationship can be an intimate and gratifying one. It's difficult, but most caregivers wouldn't have it any other way. So remember, a squeeze of the hand or an affectionate smile—or a familiar gesture or inside joke that you both share—can make your caregiver's day much easier.

Take a team approach. Try to find a way to spread caregiving responsibilities around the family, if at all possible. Let everyone play a role for which they're best suited. When my mother was sick, I was instrumental in helping everyone figure out how she could still be relatively independent: how to rearrange her house so she could stay there, and arrange transportation so she wasn't isolated at home. My brothers and my grandmother rallied to help my mom and to be there for her and for each other. It was a terrible time in our lives but in some ways it brought us all closer. If you don't have an extended family or kids at home, and one person gets saddled with all the responsibility, burnout is almost inevitable. So do whatever you can to enlist the help of nonfamily members or a paid helper to give your caregiver a break.

Caregivers need to take care of themselves. Your caregiver should follow those basic rules of life: Get plenty of sleep, eat well, and make time to exercise. Even just taking a walk can help a caregiver clear his or her head and feel refreshed. Keep an eye on your caregiver. Don't keep them at your beck and call just because you don't want to be alone. If you don't need them, send them on their way so they'll be there for you when you do need them.

Caregivers need love and support too. They need someone to talk to about what's going on—about their feelings. If a caregiver has family members around, it's easier because they can talk to one another. The stress is intense, and just being able to voice feelings of loss and frustration helps. Sharing those feelings with other people who are going through the same thing can make all the difference. If that family support is unavailable, you—as the heart patient—may have to make an extra effort to be supportive. Keeping a sense of humor and appreciating the little things that happened that day can give a caregiver solace. If you notice an interesting item in the newspaper or a funny piece on television, share it with your caregiver. Remember the golden rule: Empathize. Be mindful of the issues your caregiver faces. If something comes up, talk to each other and be as supportive and loving as you can.

A great resource for caregivers is http://www.heartmates.com. It's the only site dedicated to supporting spouses, families, and loved ones of heart patients.

How Can You Help Your Children to Cope?

How a child reacts to your heart event will depend on all kinds of factors—your child's age, personality, and sibling relationships, as well as how sick you are and the quality of your support network. The good news is your children can develop skills from this experience that can be extremely valuable in helping them to adjust to other losses and crises in life. How can you help them?

- *First, take care of yourself.* When you're on a plane, the flight attendant always instructs you to put on your own oxygen mask first, before a child's. In much the same way, you're going to have to take care of yourself first—physically and emotionally—in order to be able to take care of your child. Take your medicines, visit your doctor, reduce your risk factors, and deal with the emotional issues associated with your illness. If you're not taking care of yourself emotionally, it will be very difficult for you to be emotionally available to your kids.
- *Keep the routine as normal as possible.* Kids are adaptable, but it takes time for them to adjust to change. Your kids will feel more secure if you try to keep the family routines normal. Stick with traditional family rituals, if you can—whether that means a favorite TV show on Tuesdays or a special breakfast on Sunday mornings. That will help everyone feel more secure. Make sure the kids get to see their friends and, if at all possible, continue their extracurricular activities.

- *Answer questions concretely and clearly.* Don't elaborate unless a child indicates he or she wants more information. Adolescent children can tolerate more details. You know your child best—use your own judgment. But don't offer false reassurance. If something is seriously wrong with you, don't tell your children you'll be fine. Kids have a sixth sense—they'll know immediately if you're trying to conceal something.

- *Anticipate your child's concerns.* Watch your child's body language for signs of concern or anxiety. Some kids pick at their food, others bite their nails or twist their hair. You know your children best. If they seem nervous, clingy, or anxious, follow their cues and open the door to a conversation. Children of any age—including teenagers—may lack the developmental resources to express their concerns, which can cause them to worry and feel stress. Be alert to the signs of stress (see page 120).

- *Let kids help.* If your children show an interest in caring for you physically, by all means allow them to help. A younger child can help you by getting you a drink, a bandage, a pillow, or a blanket. The older they are, the more they can do. Helping you can make your kids feel that they've some control over the changes involving you and the family. But be careful: Don't let your kids give up their social lives or daily routines to care for you.

- *Make sure your kids don't feel guilty.* It's important to reassure your children—no matter how old they are—that they are in no way responsible for your heart disease. They might imagine that something they did or said may have caused your heart problem. Tell them in no uncertain terms that it is no one's fault. It just happened and now you're doing everything you can to make it better.

- *Listen carefully to your kids.* Again, recognize that they've experienced a loss. Encourage them to share their feelings, and try not to minimize those feelings or become defensive about the changes in your family. Just acknowledge what they feel and support them. A valuable approach to listening involves repeating back to them what they've said. That helps them see that you're really listening and ensures that you've understood them correctly. For example, you might say: "It sounds like you're a little scared," or "You seem concerned that you'll miss the soccer tournament next week."

- *Help them understand what's going on.* Try to tell your children what to expect next, including your limitations and abilities. That will help them feel more in control. Also, tell them how you feel. Sharing your own feelings lets them know that you're human, and helps them identify with their loss and the process of grieving. But remember: The purpose of sharing your feelings is to help them cope more effectively with the changes they're experiencing—not to unload on your kids.

- *Find new ways to spend time with your child.* If your physical activities are restricted or you're on bed rest, you can still play games with your kids, tell stories, read together, and watch movies or TV.

- *And give them extra love and kisses.* Your kids will need extra nurturing and affection—that means hugs and kisses. Just respect their boundaries with this, especially if they're teenagers. If you're lucky enough to live around extended family, this is a great time for your kids to spend more time with those relatives and get closer to them. That can give your children an emotional connection with others outside your immediate family, and can give you a break at the same time.

THE BIG QUESTION

Of course, the big—and often unspoken—question that underlies everyone's concerns is this: Are you going to die? If asked outright, you have no choice but to be honest. Children are astute: Don't say you're okay if you're not. But if your children ask, "When are you going to get better?" a reasonable answer might be: "I don't know. I don't have all the answers. But I'm doing everything I can to get better." Then they're going to watch how you act. If they see you making an effort to eat healthy, reduce stress, and eliminate unhealthy habits such as smoking, then they'll know you're trying. Remember: The best way to reassure your family that you're going to be okay is to have them watch you get better—day after day.

How Can You Help Your Adult Children Cope?

My daughter changed her career plans from moving to New York City to staying home in California to take care of me during my heart transplant. My son also moved his career from out of state to be home near me. They both became caregivers at ages twenty and twenty-four. They worry a lot more about me and are fearful of my future. And I feel guilty that I've had to rely on them. It's kind of like we reverse roles at times.

—Jo Beth, Alta Loma, CA, age 55

Adult children bring a different set of issues to the table, but they won't escape your heart event unscathed. Even though they've left home, you're still their mom. That means your heart event will trigger feelings of loss for them too—a loss of their old images of you, a loss of how they see you in their future, even a loss of their own youth and sense of immortality. Here are some of the issues that may arise:

- They may live a good distance away, have demanding jobs and even families of their own, so it can be difficult for them to be with you emotionally and physically. They may worry a lot about you and feel less in control of the situation because they don't live nearby. That can create stress.
- They could also have fears that they might develop your heart problem. Or, as I mentioned earlier, they may be in denial about that possibility, refusing to make lifestyle changes that you suggest (see page 119).
- Conversely, they might be angry with you for your lifestyle choices. Adult children can be your fiercest critics. If they feel you haven't changed your habits or see you breaking the rules, they can be particularly tough. Because they feel helpless and scared, they may go overboard in trying to control your behavior. That causes tremendous stress and anxiety in the relationship.
- They might not share their true feelings with you, because they're being overly protective of you and think you're unable to handle it.

- If they can, they might make major sacrifices to be near you and help you out, changing their career paths or moving a great distance. And if they live nearby, they might be actively engaged in caregiving. That represents a major role reversal and can require some adjusting.

How can you handle these situations? For starters, follow the guidelines that appear earlier in this chapter for your live-in family members. That means being affectionate and empathic, and keeping the lines of communication open. Here are some approaches that also work well:

- *To reassure your adult children,* take them with you to a doctor visit and let them ask the doctor questions in front of you. It not only makes them feel better, it gives them information and a sense of security that you're in good hands and going to be okay.
- *Make an effort at long-distance communication.* If they're out of town, write letters explaining how you feel about them and how proud you are of them. They'll find reassurance in your support and encouragement, and it will tell them that you're well enough to think about them!
- *Talk openly with them.* If they come for a visit, have a family discussion to open up the doors of communication. Talk openly about their feelings and worries—and your own. Be honest and forthright about your medical situation. But don't delve too much into specifics. It's important to set boundaries with your adult children. There's no need to tell them every sordid detail about your physical or emotional condition. They may be adults, but they're still your children; don't use them as your therapist. You want to share your feelings, but try not to burden them too much with your problems.
- *Share your concerns about their health.* Help your children to find a way to cope with their fears about their own mortality or having a heart problem by encouraging them to see a health-care provider or therapist, if needed. If they don't want to pursue it, just let them be.
- *Draw them close to you.* You might be tempted to keep them at a distance to protect them emotionally. Don't do it. Instead, find

ways to see more of them. They'll find comfort in seeing you get better and they may need the extra time with you to deal with their feelings of loss.

- *Be there for them.* If you think that your adult children are sheltering you from their problems and you want them to stop, talk to them about it. Tell them you've handled their problems since they were born and you'll continue to help them as long as they'll let you in. Reassure them that you can handle it and you'll be okay.

What Do You Do When Adult Children Are Angry about Your Lifestyle?

Say they see you smoking a cigarette or eating a bowl of ice cream. First of all, you need to be honest: tell them what you are and aren't willing to give up. You might also want to tell them that it's a step-by-step process. You're making changes, but it takes time. You might say: "I'm in a program that will help me quit smoking, but I haven't fully given it up yet. You'll have to be patient," or, with the ice cream: "There are certain things I'm not willing to give up. I'm going to have a little ice cream every day. But in every other way I'm trying to improve my eating habits. This is my one treat for the day. And I'm afraid you're going to have to accept it. It's where I am right now." It's important to draw a line. Don't let them treat you badly because of their feelings of loss or judgmental attitudes. You might understand their anger, but it's important that they not take it out on you.

How Do You Deal with Adult Children As Caregivers?

Let them be there for you. It gives them a sense of closeness to you and empowers them with some control in an abnormal situation. If they make sacrifices—like changing jobs or moving across country—recognize that it's because they want to be there for you. They love you and want to feel needed. Don't let yourself feel guilty. You took care of them when they were children; be proud that they want to help take care of you. And show your appreciation.

You know your adult child. If it seems like he or she is feeling stress or taking on too much responsibility, or they're doing far more than is necessary, you need to talk with them. If it gets to that point, tell them you're ready for more independence or that you feel able to do more things, and you don't need them full time. Encourage them to take a break. Be appreciative, but gently release them from their obligation.

THE OUTSIDE WORLD

This chapter focused on three key areas to helping your family to regain its balance—communication, empathy, and setting clear boundaries. If you approach your family in a caring, open manner, it can bring all of you closer together. In Chapter 7, I'll address issues related to your friends and society so you can begin to cope more effectively with any potential obstacles that come your way.

chapter seven

STRENGTHENING
RELATIONSHIPS

Friends and Society

Be who you are and say what you feel
because those who mind don't matter
and those who matter don't mind.

—Dr. Seuss

I love Dr. Seuss's wisdom, don't you? True friends don't mind what you do—they'll be there for you, no matter what. And when a crisis strikes, you find out fast who your true friends are. In fact, that process—of discovering who you can really count on—can be a surprisingly difficult element of your recovery. The true friends are the ones with whom you can safely share your feelings; with whom you stay in touch, even if that means just calling to say Hi; the people who are there for you no matter what's going on in their own lives or yours. They're the ones that just love and accept you for you.

Friendships shift and change throughout your life, and heart disease is one of the things that can shake up your friendships and spark a shift. Following a heart event, you may find that you're disappointed in some of your friends. What they do and don't do in response to your illness may disappoint you. Maybe it's something they say to you or about you. Maybe they just aren't able to be supportive. You can end up wondering if they were ever really your friends in the first place. All this can feel sad, even a bit tragic, because you're already experiencing a sense of loss and you're particularly vulnerable. You may find it reassuring to know that many women heart patients report that, although they lose some friends, they also gain new ones. It's all part of the shifts under way in your life.

One thing is certain: Friends really can make a difference in your re-covery and your frame of mind. In fact, studies have shown that heart pa-tients do significantly better if they have a strong social network of friends and family.[1][2][3][4] And if you don't have a partner or spouse, having a confidant, a friend to provide emotional support, is particularly impor-tant.[5] Friends can give you support and encouragement when you're struggling to change your habits or maintain a healthier lifestyle. They can join you while you exercise or eat at a healthy restaurant, and their companionship can be critical to your recovery efforts. For some people, friends might just as well be family. They provide emotional support in the form of encouragement, understanding, companionship, and just plain fun. They help you get through those rough spots, make you laugh, and listen to your troubles. During your recovery, they can also provide invaluable practical help—taking you to appointments, bringing you meals, driving your children around, and running errands. It's not sur-prising that having friends reduces stress. And as you know, reducing stress reduces the release of stress hormones, which helps prevent fur-ther damage to your heart.[6][7]

---

1. M. R. Janevic, N. K. Janz, J. A. Dodge, Y. Wang, X. H. Lin, and N. M. Clark, "Longitudinal Effects of Social Support on the Health and Functioning of Older Women with Heart Disease," *International Journal of Aging & Human Development* 59 (2004): 153–75.

2. Sotile and Cantor-Cooke, *Thriving with Heart Disease.*

3. American Psychological Association. "Research to the Heart of the Matter." *Monitor on Psychology* 32 (1)(2001).

4. N. Frasure-Smith et al., "Social Support, Depression, and Mortality During the First Year after Myocardial Infarction," *Circulation* 101 (2000): 1919–24.

5. Janevic et al., "Longitudinal Effects."

6. Sotile and Cantor-Cooke, *Thriving with Heart Disease.*

7. A. Rozanski et al., "Impact of Psychological Factors on the Pathogenesis of Cardiovascular Disease and the Implications for Therapy," *Circulation* 99 (1999): 2192–2217.

How Friendships Can Change: One Study

One survey of women with heart disease found that:

- Overall, 42 percent of the women surveyed said their relationships had changed—with half saying they had improved.
- More women reported a deterioration of their relationships with friends than with family.
- In particular, they said physical limitations or lower energy levels prevented them from spending as much time with their friends or sharing activities they used to share.
- Some felt they had less in common with their friends, some of whom couldn't understand the serious nature of the illness or were unable to sympathize with them.
- Others found their friends' increased concern for their well-being to be overly confining or controlling.
- Some said that during their illness they made new friends who, in some cases, became more valued than their old friends.

Source: Marcuccio, E, Loving, N, Bennett, SK, Hayes, SN (2003). A survey of attitudes and experiences of women with heart disease. *Women's Health Issues*, 13, 23–31.

A recent study demonstrated that Americans have one-third fewer friends than they did twenty years ago. That means people are more likely to be isolated and lonely than they used to be, and that's not good for anyone's well-being.[8] The problems associated with loneliness can be magnified for a heart patient, because sometimes friends that you've always relied on just don't come through for you in ways you expect. Friends can get frustrated about your health and not know how to help. Or a relationship can change because you have to change the way you do things in your life. Sometimes, even if friends have the best intentions, they can say and do some pretty unexpected things.

---

8. M. McPherson, L. Smith-Lovin, and M. E. Brashears, "Social Isolation in America: Changes in Core Discussion Networks over Two Decades," *American Sociological Review* (June 2006).

FRIENDSHIP BLOOPERS

Remember my astute friend who thought maybe my chest pain was "all in my head"? After my third stent was placed and I had radiation to a vessel in my heart, I became physically incapacitated because of severe chest pain. I could not walk from room to room without taking a nitroglycerin tablet. She told me that I needed medications for anxiety and depression to ease my "thoughts" about chest pain. Of course, a few weeks later, I ended up with a two-way bypass. Her inability to be supportive—and to trust my instincts—told me a lot about our friendship. The relationship has never been the same, in part because she never apologized or acknowledged the error in her judgment.

Unfortunately I'm not alone. It's not uncommon to lose friends to your heart disease—or, at least, to feel you've lost your friends. Many women experience feelings of isolation and estrangement from people they trusted.

> *I often feel and have experienced being secluded and distanced from many of my friends (and some family). I've always been very independent but with this—it's made me even lonelier and sadder than independent. Nowadays I feel I have to depend on others as well as myself to get me through this and sometimes there is no one there.*
>
> —Sarah, West Hempstead, NY, age 29

This experience is not unlike what some women go through when they're getting a divorce. Friends fall away because they're afraid they might catch the same disease. After all, if it can happen to you, it can happen to them.

> *My friends have been a source of support but it is kind of like, "You have heart disease and I don't. Therefore, I don't have to think about this or what you're going through." Sometimes I think I'm a threat to them because they can see what can happen to them and they don't want to face all that.*
>
> —Diana, Des Moines, IA, age 55

It's not hard to tell when a friend is uncomfortable with the situation. She no longer seems to know how or what to say to you, and there's an air of awkwardness between the two of you that never existed before. You can sense a friend's discomfort. Maybe she stops coming by or calling. Or if you start talking about your heart disease, she's quiet and says nothing at all. Reactions like these can be difficult and put a strain on the friendship.

Sometimes friendships change because you no longer share the same activities due to your physical limitations or changes in your interests. Maybe you've had to stop going to aerobics classes, running with the neighborhood joggers, or hanging out at the local pool. This can have a big impact on relationships that were once anchored in those activities.

> *I used to exercise with my friend all the time and then I had a heart attack. I decided to change my exercise routine, which benefited my cardiac health. At first she seemed to support the change, but then she stopped calling me and we didn't do anything else together to maintain the friendship. Now I barely see her and we rarely talk. The change in our relationship really has been hurtful to me.*
>
> —Kim, Atlanta, GA, age 42

Sometimes, without even realizing it, your friend sees changes in you, and she may not understand or accept those changes. Painfully, she might distance herself from you. Feelings can get hurt and relationships become scarred. In fact, these experiences with friends can be quite difficult to deal with—for both you and your friend.

HANDLING FRIENDSHIPS

> *One who looks for a friend without faults will have none.*
>
> —Hasidic Saying

Accept your friends' limitations. Women heart patients have to learn to accept limitations—even flaws—they may not have noticed before. Maybe your friend is preoccupied with her own life, and not in a position to offer genuine help and support. Maybe she's trying to help, but you notice she's being bossy with your kids or judgmental with you. Whatever it may be, those limitations may always have been there and it's possible that you just never personally experienced them before. We all have flaws. Try to be as forgiving and accepting as you can be. If you want to put some distance between yourself and a friend for a while, feel free to do so. But it doesn't have to be permanent. Many enduring friendships have ebbs and flows.

Don't expect too much.   You might reach an impasse in a friendship because you're expecting too much from your friend. In the previous chapter, I talked about the importance of communicating your needs to your family and not expecting them to automatically know exactly what you need from them. The same holds true of your friends. They may not know how to help. They may not be fully capable of dealing with their own feelings about your illness and the lifestyle changes you have to make. They may feel frightened, awkward, or uncomfortable. They may have something going on in their own lives right now—and not want to burden you with it. Don't let their absence or shortcomings cause feelings of disappointment and a sense of isolation. Talk to your friends. Stay in touch with them. Remember: They might be waiting to hear from you. If you make an effort and don't hear back from them, try to let it go. Remember: Their reactions may have nothing to do with you.

Sometimes it's your friend's problem—not yours.   Generally friends have good intentions, but at times their reactions or behavior towards you may seem indifferent, unsupportive, and lacking in empathy. Here's an example:

> *I called my friend and told her that I was going to give a talk to a group of women about heart disease. I told her that I wanted to help other women to not go through what I've been through. Her first reaction was silence. Then she said, "Well, I guess you're one of those people who just loves to stay busy. You know Joy, everyone has something or another wrong with them." And I thought to myself: Does she not hear herself?*
>
> —Joy, Livermore, CA, age 48

Joy's smart enough to recognize the problem is not hers. A friend who fails to give you support and encouragement is likely to have her own emotional issues. Maybe Joy's friend is jealous of her courage and not happy that she has to share Joy with her new passion. Or she's angry with Joy that she won't let the "heart disease focus" just drop. Maybe Joy's friend feels guilty that she doesn't devote much of her own life to helping others. Whatever the reason, this is her friend's bag of troubles—not Joy's. So Joy has learned to think twice before sharing such information with this particular friend in the future.

TAKE A FRIENDSHIP INVENTORY

Becoming a heart patient catapults you into a place where you recognize your own mortality. This is the time in your life to embrace the things that give you joy and weed out the things that are unfulfilling. Friendships are no different. Part of your healing and recovery can be aided by taking an inventory of your friendships. Some friendships develop because you grew up together or went to the same school. Others spring from a common interest. Maybe you went to the same church or synagogue, or you get together because of your kids. You might serve on the same committee, work together, or see each other at the gym. Over time these relationships either deepen or gel, or they don't. At a certain point, it's valuable to step back and determine which relationships to maintain and which to let go. Sometimes a heart event can be a watershed—a time to ask yourself which friendships are the ones that you value the most and which ones need to end. Following a heart event, there's no room in your life for unsupportive relationships. A simple rule of thumb: If someone tends to make you feel bad, strongly consider walking away from the relationship.

Unhealthy friendships.   At some point, everyone encounters people they think are their friends, but they're not. They may be delightful and entertaining, but the better you get to know them, the more obvious it becomes: They're demanding, self-centered and unable to provide the support you might need in a crisis. Oddly enough, it may take time to recognize their flaws; you might think someone is a great friend, but then the problematic nature of the friendship surfaces. Here are some characteristics such people tend to share:

- They only talk about themselves and can't seem to empathize with you. They really aren't listening.

- They can be very critical and judgmental. Nothing you do is ever good enough.
- They gossip and talk about other people behind their backs.
- They are possessive. So they have difficulty tolerating your other friends. In fact, they tend to criticize your friends.
- They are demanding—calling frequently when they need you. But they're unable to offer support when you need them.
- They may be moody and unpredictable—happy one minute and then sullen and sad the next.

Some women fall into friendships with difficult people and then, when it becomes obvious that these are not supportive and healthy friends, they find a way to disentangle themselves. For whatever reason, other women find it harder to let go of unhealthy friendships or may even be drawn to them. Following a heart event, the flaws in such relationships quickly become obvious. These are the kind of people who are genuinely incapable of offering you the support you need.

> *I had a friend—or let me say, I thought she was a friend—who turned on me when I had my heart attack and then my bypass surgery. At first, she'd show up at the hospital, but all she'd do was talk about herself. She never asked me anything about how I was feeling. Once I got home, I had to take care of my own needs at that time and change my habits, so I was less available to her neediness and demands. She couldn't seem to get what she needed from the relationship with me, so she stopped calling me. If I see her in public, she won't even acknowledge that I'm there. Now that I'm better, I see how emotionally unhealthy she really is.*
>
> —Sandy, Toledo, OH, age 37

If you have a friend who fits this description, for your peace of mind, think about whether the friendship is in your best interest. You might find that this is the best time to let go of such a friendship. Some things to consider are:

- Ending this relationship shows your commitment to taking care of yourself.

- You've had a heart event. You need to be true to yourself and your feelings.
- Life is too short to be in an unhappy friendship. You deserve better.
- Get help by talking about your feelings to clergy or a therapist. Try to use this as an opportunity to understand why you picked a friend like this, so you can avoid these types of relationships in the future.

Lifestyle friends. Sometimes following a heart event, you'll lose friends because you're changing your lifestyle habits to stay healthy. Generally, the best approach is simple: Just let them go.

> *Friends? Gosh, this is an easy one. I have none of the friends now that I had prior to my heart attack. A couple of reasons for this, I suppose, is I could no longer hang out with the group who would run to smoke when things got tough in the office, and I would no longer go out for the cocktail hour after work. Actually, some of them have not spoken to me since I had my heart attack. I don't know why and now I really don't care why. I have real friends now, the ones who stepped in when the others ran out. I'm truly blessed to have the friends who are in my life today.*
>
> —Tasha, Hot Springs, AR, age 40

Foul weather friends. After a crisis such as a heart event, people seem to come out of the woodwork. It may seem like the entire community has descended upon your family to help. But that can be a mixed blessing. Relationships that you thought were long gone can come back to haunt you. And suddenly people you feel you barely know are there to lend their support. It can feel awkward and leave you wondering, Who are these people? What are they doing here? Do they really care about me? Well, honestly, all I can say is: It doesn't really matter. They've come to help you and your family in a time of need. No matter how strange these sudden outbursts of friendship make you feel, just try to appreciate them. Don't worry. Most people are just helping out to be friendly or neighborly. As soon as you begin to recover, most of them will disappear again.

But you might be in for a surprise. Some of these people might end up being a bigger part of your life than you expected. So just let these friendships run their natural course. Over time you'll find out whether any of them will be valuable and lasting relationships, just as you would with any other friendship.

A Friendship Pyramid

When it hurts to look back, and you're scared to look ahead, you can look beside you and your best friend will be there.

—Anonymous

Years ago, a wise colleague of mine shared an idea with me: It can be helpful, she said, to view your friendships in a pyramid formation. I've since used this approach with many patients and they do find it helpful. Look at it this way: At the very pointy top of the pyramid are your very best friends—that may be one or two people. On the level below that are your good friends—you probably have a few more of those. Below that are your other friends and acquaintances; there may be a lot of people in this group, but you may not know them too well or see them too often. Here's how they all stack up.

Best friends.   These are your closest friends, the ones who are there for you whenever you need them, who reciprocate your feelings, and invest time and energy in the relationship. Aside from your immediate family, these are the people who know you the best. They're probably the friends who've known you the longest. And, not surprisingly, they're the friends that can give you the most support following a heart event.

One of my best friends lives in Virginia. She was so upset by my bypass surgery that she kept insisting that she was going to come to Memphis to stay with me. She was disappointed when I told her not to come. But she would have been here in an instant if I'd given her the okay. She called often, giving me the kind of emotional support that only a close friend can provide. She sent me sweet Get Well cards in the mail and she gave me an invaluable gift: She made me laugh. Friends like her don't grow on trees! Be grateful for your dearest friends. That's all you really need to do. Just accept and appreciate the fact that they're there for you.

Of course, sometimes your best friend can be your toughest critic and adviser, the person who forces you to face reality before you're quite ready. Maybe she's insisting that you quit smoking. Or she brings you a fantastic diet book before you're emotionally prepared to take on a diet. She might be the first person to identify a mental-health issue—such as depression or anxiety—before you recognize it, and encourage you to get help. That's because your best friend loves you. So, if she says the wrong thing, cut her some slack. And, if she pushes too hard, recognize that she's only trying to help you get better.

> *My best friend and biggest supporter of my growth is the one who challenges me to face the things I don't want to see. And to her I give thanks!*
>
> —Susan, Mission Viejo, CA, age 58

You're lucky if you have a friend who's able to really nurture you during your recovery. Someone who knows what you need even if you don't realize it yourself, who is available and emotionally capable of providing you with genuine support. With a friend like this, you can accept the fact that she's there for you when you're sick or emotionally troubled because you know the tides will change. And when they do, you'll be there for her. Of course, a best friend isn't keeping score.

FROM ONE BEST FRIEND TO ANOTHER

Your heart disease has only affected me in that I realize how valuable you are to me and how fragile our time really is . . . that I could have lost you at any moment and how devastating that would have been. Your heart disease has made me realize how much closer it has brought you to your own mortality and how much more value you place on God, love, time, friends and family (not that you didn't before, but it's much more obvious now). All in all, since you are still here with us, your heart disease has been, as funny as it sounds a good thing. Beautiful things have come from it.

—Ashley's Friend, Phoenix, AZ, age 48

My closest friend was an invaluable support to both my husband and me. She was there in the days immediately following my by-pass surgery. She took me to follow-up appointments. Each time I had a stent implanted, she was there to provide support and com-fort. She even acted as a kind of interpreter when I couldn't ask questions that needed to be asked or process information that was being given to me. A surprising result of my heart disease is that we've become much closer.

—Mary, Cortlandt Manor, NY, age 54

Good friends.   At the next level of the pyramid are your good friends. These are people you feel you can talk to—but maybe not about everything. You probably haven't known them as long or don't know them as well as your best friends. It may be that you know them in one particular arena of your life—like through work or your kids. You trust them and value their friend-ship, but the emotional connection just isn't as strong. So you're likely to expect a little less of one another than you do of your best friends.

Good friends can be a bit harder to predict when you're in the middle of a crisis. In fact, they might say or do some surprising things following your heart event. They can act awkward, uncomfortable, and uncertain. They may not have a clue about what to say to you or how to be supportive.

This is a hard place to be with your friends and it can make you feel isolated and alone. Some of these friendships will change because of your heart event. That can be particularly painful, because it can feel like another loss. Why does it happen? For one thing, illness inspires inti-macy. Sometimes, when people visit you in the hospital or in your bed-room, or even in your home, they are seeing you in a completely new setting. The attention is often focused on you and how you feel, and very personal subjects related to your health and your emotional well-being. These conditions can really test a friendship if you haven't been through much together. One of the biggest issues that comes up with good friends is trying to gauge just how close you can get—how much you can share and how much you can expect from them. Here are a few issues that can arise:

- *Confidentiality.* When you're sick, you want to be able to talk about how you're doing and feeling without having it spread all over the community. Because once the word gets out that you're having a procedure or something's wrong, everyone you know will call about the news. So you don't want friends who repeat everything you tell them. How will you know if it's safe to share your feelings about your heart disease with your good friends? Share information with your good friends only if you're completely comfortable doing so. Use your judgment about your relationship and decide exactly what's safe to share and when.

- *Comfort level.* Not all your good friends will be equally comfortable talking about your medical condition. Take statements like, "They did an angiogram and angioplasty today that showed . . ." or, "I feel good, but my doctor wants to do more tests," or even "My scar is causing me discomfort." A best friend knows you well enough to feel completely at ease with such comments. But a good friend may not handle it quite so readily. It might be too personal. How do you decide who can handle what? Take your cues from your friends. Watch and listen—and ask yourself: How did she react to what I said? Did she recoil or lack empathy? Did she seem uncomfortable? Did she not respond at all? You'll know which friends to keep at a comfortable distance by observing their behavior.

- *Empathy and support.* Not all your good friends will be good at being supportive and caring when you're recovering or in the months that follow. It may be because that's not who they are; or because you're not that close to each other; or for any number of other reasons, including their own fears. You'll learn over time who you can and can't talk to about the ongoing issues related to your heart disease. Observe your friends when you turn to them for support, and ask yourself: Was she a good listener? Did she come back with a supportive response? Or was she dismissive or unresponsive? Did she just draw a blank, or maybe even turn the discussion towards herself? Based on the answers to these questions, you'll know which of your good friends are capable of being there for you emotionally and who you can safely share intimate information with in the future.

Acquaintances. At the lowest level of the pyramid are your acquaintances. These might be your neighbors, coworkers, or people you see around town throughout your week. They might be friends you see in social situations, but you're not particularly close. Conversations with acquaintances don't generally get too far or go too deep. In normal everyday life, the boundaries are pretty clear. Unfortunately, when you have an illness, those boundaries break down. Suddenly people with whom you've never had a single intimate conversation are asking about something that's very intimate: your heart event and your recovery.

Their interest and concern may be genuine, but it can be awkward. Sometimes it can feel a bit like voyeurism. You may feel as if your privacy is being invaded or you're being accosted with inappropriate questions. Other times it can become difficult, because people are asking very personal questions, but the nature of the relationship requires very superficial answers. If you begin to tell them actual details about your illness, they quickly grow uncomfortable—after all, they barely know you. As a result, the process itself can be stressful.

> *Many of my church friends frequently make the comment that they are glad that I'm no longer ill. They think this way because I don't look sick. I have quit reminding them that heart failure is chronic and progressive. I've learned just to let their comments slide past me.*
>
> —Susan, Mission Viejo, CA, age 58

The best way to deal with acquaintances is to keep these discussions as simple and superficial as possible. Generic comments such as, "I appreciate your concern" or, "Thanks for asking—I'm much better," always work best with acquaintances. If you tell them the truth or share too much information, it's quite possible they'll become embarrassed or tune you out. If you tell them to mind their own business—and sometimes you'll wish you could—you'll embarrass yourself by being too abrupt. Remember: They're not doing anything wrong, no matter how irritating it may feel to be questioned about your health every time you see them. It may help to know it happens to all of us—so try not to let it get to you. And keep an open mind. Sometimes, as this process unfolds, acquaintances can actually become friends.

What Can You Do about Overprotective Friends?

Two of my good friends treat me like I am a fragile child, which I find
extremely smothering. I told them to back off and give me my space.
—Susan, Mission Viejo, CA, age 58

Just as it affects your family, your illness can make your friends feel helpless and scared. They're afraid that something might happen to you. They don't want to lose you. And with those feelings come a need to control the uncontrollable—to mother and nurture you because that's the way they feel they can really help. But this treatment can grate on you. How do you deal with it?

Approach them gently.   Create a clear path of communication with these friends. Tell them you appreciate how much they care about you. Tell them how you feel. But do so with gentleness, humor, and sensitivity.

Explain that it makes you uncomfortable.   Friends are typically on an equal footing—adult to adult. If your friends are treating you as fragile, then it becomes more like a parent/child relationship, which puts you in a child role. That's unfulfilling and problematic in friendships. Let your friends know that when they treat you with kid gloves it changes the nature of the relationship in ways that make you uncomfortable.

Reassure them.   Address their underlying fears by telling them what you're actively doing to improve your health. Remind them that you're making these changes within your own time frame. Sometimes your friends just need to hear that you're going to be okay for them to feel more comfortable with the relationship. Being open and honest with your closest friends reassures them. It really helps if you tell your friends that you're still you, that they can be themselves around you, and that you're not fragile like an uncooked egg. Sometimes you need to state the obvious to get your friends to feel more at ease.

I reduced the fear for my friends by educating them as I became
educated about heart disease. I'm a survivor. I'm strong. They can

*still lean on me. I've got lots of hugs. I don't break. I love them all
and want us to grow old together. That means staying strong and
healthy together! I'm not alone in this and neither are they.*
                                   —Ellen, Beverly Hills, MI, age 53

Steer your conversations in a new direction.   Most heart patients get very
tired of being asked, "How are you doing? How are you feeling today?"
every time they see their friends.

> *My friends are scared. I know I look good and even perhaps better
> than I once did. But I wish they'd keep those stares and ridicu-
> lously loaded statements of "How are you feeling?" followed by
> "Are you sure?" to themselves. It's stressful on our friendship to
> feel as if you're being constantly watched.*
>   —Billie, Las Vegas, NV, age 44

Billie's problem couldn't be more common. It gets old answering these
types of questions and tilts your relationship in an unnatural direction.
Just say: "Let's not focus on my health today. Let's talk about something
else." Of course, this will create an awkward gap in the conversation and
it'll be your job to fill it. Ask them something about their lives.

What To Do about A Friend Who Gossips

Everybody knows people who gossip—and, interestingly enough, everyone seems to know exactly who the people who gossip are. Doubtless,
you know a few of them.

So what do you do if you have heart disease, want to maintain your privacy, and have a friend who's a gossip? Unfortunately, you may have to decide whether this is a friend worth keeping. After all, it's hard work not
being able to be open and share with your friends. It leaves you feeling as if
you have to keep a screen up when you talk and filter what you say to her.

But what if this friend has a great sense of humor—and that really
cheers you up? Or she's wonderful with your kids and has a tremen-
dously generous spirit? Or you've been friends forever. Just be selective
about what you share with her. Don't provide her with details about your
health—because you know she'll repeat it and you could end up getting
ten phone calls from mutual acquaintances. Just be careful what you say.

THE WONDERFUL WOMEN IN MY CIRCLE

When I was little, I used to believe in the concept of one best friend, and then I started to become a woman and found out that if you allow your heart to open up, God will show you the best in many friends.

- One friend is needed when you're going through things with your man.
- Another friend is needed when you're going through things with your mom.
- Another is needed when you want to shop, share, heal, hurt, or joke.
- One friend will say let's pray together, another let's cry together, another let's fight together or another let's walk away together.
- One friend will meet your spiritual needs. Other friends will share your shoe fetish, your love for movies, another will be with you during a time of confusion, another will be a friend who clarifies for you, and another friend will be the wind beneath your wings.
- But whatever their assignment in your life, on whatever the occasion, on whatever the day, or whenever you need them, those are your best friends.

—Anonymous

Of course, if you have a friend who's a gossip, you may well have learned that lesson already.

HOW TO HOLD ONTO YOUR FRIENDS

Heart disease can be a lifelong issue and it's difficult to know how to balance your friends' needs with your own. Let's face it—heart disease changes us. And it can throw any friendship into a bit of a spin. For one thing, your friends can feel exhausted by listening to you share your feelings and concerns about heart disease. It can make them feel helpless and frustrated. Or they might just grow tired of it. Here are some things you can do to keep your friendships healthy.

Balance the conversation. To keep the relationship fresh and rewarding for both of you, you need to find ways to balance the conversation. Remember:

Your friends have lives of their own and may be going through something as well. It might not be as dramatic as your illness, but it may be just as significant to them. Having balanced communications with your friends means thinking about where they are emotionally. If the conversation is always about you, the friendship is bound to suffer. So ask them: What's new? What's going on? How are things at work? How are the kids?

Change the subject.   Talk about anything besides your health—a book you're reading, a great movie, your kids, the weather, your favorite soap opera. If a friend turns the conversation to your health every time you see her, remind her that your relationship can't thrive if the focus is always about your health—that you don't want to think about your health issues all the time and she probably doesn't either. She might appreciate getting the relationship back to a more normal footing.

Practice listening.   It's a rare and skilled friend who knows when to listen and when to talk. But listening will help you understand what's going on in your friends' lives, so you can continue to be a friend to them. And it can give you valuable information about your relationship. Does it seem like they're scared about your health and well-being? Are they uncomfortable talking with you? If you're listening, you're in a much better position to address their real concerns.

Don't be preachy.   When you get diagnosed with heart disease, it's not uncommon to educate yourself about it. You begin to think of yourself as an expert. Just try not to be the missionary who tries to convert your friends to the truth about heart-healthy behavior. That can be a turnoff in a friendship; it can make your friends uncomfortable and create resentment. After all, no one likes to be lectured to.

> *I try very hard not to preach to my friends. And I don't point out things that they do that are not heart healthy, although sometimes I want to. I will share new information with my friends if the issue comes up. But if they choose not to take my advice, I try not to get angry when they don't listen.*
>
> —Diana, Des Moines, IA, age 55

Never give medical advice. It's one thing if your friends ask for your opinion or information based on your experience. But it's very important for you not to give medical advice no matter how well educated you are about heart disease. Leave that up to the health-care providers.

Be appreciative. Friendships come and go over the course of your life. You move or your marital status changes. Maybe you have children but your friend doesn't. Or you have an empty nest and you work, but your friend doesn't. Even so, some friendships are worth fighting for—those are the relationships that you know in your heart are meant to last. Make sure you nurture those friendships. Be grateful. Be thoughtful. Be thankful. And take time to be with your dearest friends.

TAKE TIME FOR FRIENDSHIPS

Life is busy. And when you're adapting to all the changes that come with heart disease, it can be even more challenging to maintain your friendship. Your friends are important to your health. So don't shortchange them. Here are some ways to make sure you sustain your important friendships.

- Actively schedule time to be together. You can volunteer, join a club, or a promote a cause together.
- Consciously make an effort to stay connected by phone, letter, or e-mail.
- Create shared time together. Commit to do an exercise class, an adult education class, or a book club with one another.
- Plan ahead. Buy tickets to the symphony or theater together.
- Talk to each other openly about time constraints and responsibilities.
- Make time alone without partners or children.
- Be thoughtful and considerate of your friend's needs. Ask your friend when there's a convenient time for her to talk or to get together with you.
- You can just have your friend come over for a glass of wine, a cup of tea, or to just chat. You don't always have to do something to be together.

Treasure your friendships that are anchored in history. Those friendships remind us of where we came from. If an old friend is far away, make an extra effort. Plan a trip or vacation together.

How to Make New Friends

With all of the transitions that most women go through in life there are always times when women need to make new friends. Women heart patients are no exception. Where do you start? First, realize that to make new friends you have to put yourself out there by taking risks with women you meet. Here are some tips:

- Be assertive with new people. Talk to them, smile, and see how the conversation flows.
- Make yourself available to others by using positive body language. Say hello and start up the conversation. Introduce yourself.
- You can meet potential new friends at your exercise class, at work, at a book club, at your kids' school, or at your church or synagogue.
- You might have to be the one who reaches out to initiate the relationship. Start by inviting women you meet and feel comfortable with to lunch, to get a cup of coffee, or to take a walk.
- Recognize that relationships take time. Don't put too much pressure on a potential new friend. They may begin to think of you as too needy and worry that you'll take up too much of their already limited time.
- If you get rejected in your efforts to make a friend, try not to take it personally. Brush off the feelings and move on to the next potential friend. In the long run, your efforts will be worthwhile.
- Just remember that friendships take time, energy, and mutual experiences to develop. Try to be patient. It will happen.

Friendships are incredibly important to women heart patients for their overall recovery and well-being. Friends help shape who we are and through those relationships we learn about the complicated nature of others, our needs, feelings, and ourselves. Strengthening your friendships takes hard work and energy. But friends are worth it. When it comes to friends, don't sell yourself short by accepting less than you deserve. Get rid of the bad apples and hold onto the good ones, because they're a godsend.

BRANCHING OUT

In Part 3, we move from focusing on rebuilding your sense of self to dealing with the outside world. Chapter 8 looks at how to manage your work life without fear of reprisals, how to protect your rights, and how to make effective and healthy work-related choices. What are the issues that arise when you go back to work? That's coming up next.

PART THREE

NEGOTIATING THE OUTER WORLD

I could not, at any age,
be content to take my place
by the fireside and simply look on.
Life was meant to be lived.
Curiosity must be kept alive.
One must never, for whatever reason,
turn his back on life.

—Eleanor Roosevelt

chapter eight

MANAGING YOUR WORK LIFE

Facing the Challenge

Choose a job you love, and you will
never have to work a day in your life.
—Confucius

Heart disease has tentacles that seem to touch every aspect of a patient's life, including her job. Following a heart event, some women can just get out of the hospital and keep working at the same job in the same way without any problems. But for many heart patients it's not quite that simple.

Many heart patients find they must reduce their hours, if only temporarily, and ease back into full-time employment. Others find that it's time to make a change. Maybe their jobs are just too stressful or demanding, or they have difficulties with their coworkers or boss when they return to work. For some, a heart event provides an opportunity to reflect on what's important to them, and that process inspires them to change their job or career, or even to retire early. Of course, there are also women who are no longer able to work because of their heart disease. In this chapter, we'll explore all these possibilities and how to cope with them.

TOO MUCH, TOO FAST

I'll never forget a conversation I had with a man who called me after he'd seen a magazine article about my experience and whose wife, Mary, had just had a heart attack. She was about forty years old, a lawyer in a high-powered law firm, and he was very concerned because she was on the computer and telephone working with clients from her hospital bed. It seems Mary was also refusing to talk about the heart attack or how she might have to change her life once she went home. Her husband was upset and scared, unsure of where to turn. I suggested that Mary might be in shock and denial about the entire event, and I advised him to wait a little while and see whether she would start facing the realities of what might lie ahead. Seemingly she'd gone into a crisis mode and was trying to alleviate her anxiety by focusing on her work. Maybe it gave her a sense of control. Maybe she was worried that she would fall behind in her work or her partners would find out she'd had a heart attack and she'd lose her job. Or maybe she was just trying to prove to herself that she was still capable and that nothing had changed.

After that one conversation, I never found out what happened to Mary—and whether she was able to scale back in order to be healthier. But I do know that, for many heart patients, it takes time to recognize all the implications of the illness. And for some, stress can be a major issue.

During the days leading up to my heart attack, I was working extremely long hours at an intensely stressful job. I worked for a VP of a large health-care organization. The woman who was my boss was a machine; she never got tired and everything had to be perfect. She wouldn't let me take off for my birthday because we were working on a project. I worked from 7:30 one morning until 4 A.M. the next! I was beyond exhausted. Then on that same day I got into an argument with another VP in the office and started to cry hysterically. The nurses checked me out and then sent me home to rest. A few hours later my boss called me at home. She was going over things we still needed to do and giving me orders. A few minutes after I hung up, I suffered a heart attack. Since then, my health has never been the same. I have no doubt that the stress of my job led to my heart attack.

—Rachel, Jamaica, NY, age 52

Work-related stress isn't good for your health. Studies show that demanding jobs are linked to elevated blood pressure, a release of stress hormones into the bloodstream, an increase in heart rate, and an increase

ASK YOURSELF: IS MY JOB TOO STRESSFUL?

- Do you have trouble getting up in the morning to go to work?
- Do you obsess about all of the things you have to do when you get there?
- Do you have anxious feelings about work even before you walk in the door, such as butterflies, shallow breathing, and excess perspiration. Do you feel your heart racing?
- Do you feel overwhelmed more often than not by all of the work you do?
- Do you go home feeling worried about all of the unfinished things you haven't done?
- Do you snap at others at work, even your boss?
- Do you go home and feel unfulfilled and dissatisfied with your work?
- Are your work hours incompatible with the rest of your life?

If you answered "yes" to three or more of the above questions, you may want to assess whether your job is really right for you and your health.

in the size of the left ventricle of the heart.[1] Other studies show that reducing the demands of a job to average levels can reduce the risk of heart disease.[2] These facts should encourage women heart patients to look closely at the stress inherent in their jobs before returning to work.

MAKING A CHANGE

Your doctor will tell you if and when it's okay for you to go back to work, but it's up to you to decide whether you need to make a change. Having a brush with your own mortality gives you permission to review all aspects of your life including your career. Ask yourself:

---

1. P. A. Landsbergis, S. J. Schurman, B. A. Israel, et al., "Job Stress and Heart Disease: Evidence and Strategies for Prevention," *Scientific Solutions* (Summer 1993).

2. E. D. Eaker, L. M. Sullivan, M. Kelly-Hayes, et al., "Does Job Strain Increase the Risk for Coronary Heart Disease or Death in Men and Women?" *American Journal of Epidemiology* 159 (2004): 950–58.

- Is my career satisfying and fulfilling?
- Does my job reduce or increase the stress in my life?
- Was I considering some kind of job or career change before my heart event?
- Is it possible for me to change jobs?
- What are my financial constraints? Can I afford to reduce my hours or switch to a part-time job?
- Does it make sense for me to stop working altogether? Am I in a position to retire early?

Clearly your decision about work will be based on many factors, including your age, stage in life, family situation, doctor's recommendations, medical condition, and financial options. But it's important to take this moment as an opportunity to look at all the demands in your life and figure out what, if anything, needs to change. And that includes your work life. For some women, a heart event represents a powerful wake-up call.

I quit my job because I realized that the high level of stress it brought me was the biggest danger to my well-being. Now I make more time for myself and make sure that my health is the best that it can be. I enjoy life's simple pleasures so much more, such as sunny days, walks with the dog, and digging up the dirt in my flowerbeds.

—Ellen, Beverly Hills, MI, age 53

Ellen could afford to stop working. But for many women heart patients, not working isn't an option. And for many of those who must work, the issue of flexibility takes on a whole new meaning.

Being the wife of a much older, retired college professor, and caretaker of a ninety-year-old mother, and mother to two teenage sons, I had been working as a substitute teacher. This allowed me a certain amount of flexibility. After my first heart attack and surgery I got lots of support from the local schools. Basically I got to call the shots about when I wanted to work. I also was given keys to back doors and elevators to make my access to the classroom easier.

—Linda, DeKalb, IL, age 53

Many women heart patients find that they want to try to have flexibility in their work. It makes it easier to manage the rest of their lives more effectively, and enables them to reduce stress. Both of these factors—flexibility and reduced stress—are directly connected to high levels of job satisfaction. In fact, research shows that just switching to a job that's easier to manage and more convenient can improve overall job satisfaction.[3]

Whatever your reason is for deciding to make a job change—low satisfaction, high stress, or just the desire to try something new—you'll want to brainstorm to discover what options you have. Here are some possibilities:

- You can continue working full time in a different job.
- You can go back to work part time, negotiate a more flexible arrangement in your current job, or find a new, part-time job.
- Maybe you can work from your home. Or you might decide to start your own business.
- You might think about going back to school for training in another field or to enhance the skills you have. Taking Adult Education classes at a nearby college or community center can help you to decide which options are best for you.
- You might decide to stop working or retire early. Or in the long run you might decide to work in a different way altogether by volunteering.

SHIFTING PRIORITIES

A year and a half after my diagnosis, I left corporate America and all the stress behind that came with raising a family of four children while traveling for work. Now my focus is on the family. Being with, and for, the kids is the greatest job in my life—not a stress-free job by any means, as you know, but still the most wonderful days I've lived.

—Elizabeth, Plymouth, MN, age 45

---

3. D. W. Pitts, E. M. Jarry, V. M. Wilkins, and S. K. Pandey, "What Do Women Want? Men, Women, and Job Satisfaction in the Public Service," Georgia State University, Andrew Young School of Policy Studies Research Paper Series 2006, Working Paper 06-34.

Look inside yourself and really think about what matters to you the most. Weigh your options and how those options will affect you physically and emotionally. If you're like Mary, the high-powered attorney you met earlier in this chapter, ask yourself: Do I still need to be the professional who clamors to be at the top of my firm? Or can I be satisfied in a less intense job that will reduce stress—and give me more time to do other things that bring me happiness, like spending time with my children or grandchildren? Many women heart patients find that they've changed, that their idea of what offers them fulfillment is not the same as it was before their heart event.

Given what you've been through, you've been reminded of your own mortality and that life is precious. Over time, you'll reflect on all that you've experienced—all those feelings—the loss and recovery of a sense of self; the loss of your invincibility and acceptance of your own mortality; and a renewed sense of purpose. You'll come to recognize and take pride in your own strength, your capacity for survival and your ability to adapt to all these changes. That's what being a survivor is all about—and shifting your priorities is a part of that process. Try to view a job or career change as part of that process—as a new opportunity, a door opening—and a symptom of your ability to adapt to change and create a new life for yourself.

It's important to realize that resetting your priorities takes time—it's a sign of your recovery, your growth. Be patient with yourself. You may have to take small steps to make changes, but it will happen. And if it's what you want, it's doable—but it's not always easy.

After my sudden cardiac arrest, I stayed home for four months— and couldn't drive for six months. Before that, I'd had the perfect job coordinating a brand new federal grant for an urban school district. I worked half time and set my own hours. I could work and be with my kids. But because of my absence, I lost that job. When they offered me a full-time teaching position, I said no. I wouldn't have had control of my schedule. I quit because I wanted to be home with my kids. I decided that because my boys almost lost their mother, I didn't want to work full time. Four years later, my boys—now eight and eleven—are still my prior-

ity. I do part-time projects when I can, but I just don't have the perfect job anymore.

—Natasha, Lake Elmo, MN, age 38

Making career decisions can have emotional consequences. Not surprisingly, you may experience a sense of loss when you give up a job. (See the Stages of Grief in Chapter 2.) Even when your priorities are clear, you may struggle with how to strike a balance between your priorities and your financial needs. If you're grappling with these issues, I encourage you to get support from the people around you or seek counseling if you need it (see Chapter 3).

GOING BACK TO WORK

My office has been great through everything. The Congressman has supported me from the time I've been at Stanford Hospital, through my ICD (implantable cardioverter defibrillator) and pacemaker surgeries. He sat with me in the ER in Washington, D.C., after an episode, so he has been most understanding. The rest of the staff has been a great support. They ask about the doctors appointments and are an ear to listen when needed. We recently moved offices and they were conscious of the fact that we were moving into a second floor, and made sure there was an elevator for the bad days when I might not feel up to the stairs.

—Margaret, Fresno, CA, age 36

When your doctor tells you you're ready to go back to work, it feels great at first. You'll be doing something useful and productive—and, ideally, something that you enjoy. It'll get your mind off of your heart problems. Things will start getting back to normal and you'll be less worried about money because you'll be earning a living again.

But you just may have to get past a few hurdles and deal with a few issues, including your own attitudes and those of your coworkers.

Coming out. For many heart patients, the first hurdle involves telling your boss and coworkers about your heart event. It's not unusual to fear the potential consequences. Coming out about your heart illness creates legitimate concerns about how it will affect your livelihood. Can they fire you? Will you be passed by for promotion? Will your coworkers worry about you all the time? Will they treat you differently? It's scary to tell others at work because it seems that you have no control over how they will react and in turn how those reactions will make you feel.

I'll never forget Sarah, a woman I met through my association with WomenHeart. A nurse in charge of her state's public health department, Sarah's job involved getting the word out to the community about heart disease in women. That's how we met. So imagine my surprise when she told me that she'd just had a heart attack but hadn't told anyone at work yet. Sarah was afraid of the potential fallout. She knew she could still do her job well, and even though her job was a demanding one, she still loved it—and she was scared of the possibility of losing it. She was also in charge of her area, and she feared her employees would see her as a weak link, someone who could no longer pull her own weight. She thought they might feel sorry for her or think they'd have to handle her with kid gloves.

Sarah and I talked about her predicament over the phone, and just a few minutes into the conversation, she realized she had no choice—she had to tell them. For one thing, she knew that it would be potentially disastrous if she had a heart event at work and her employees didn't know about her condition. But just as importantly, Sarah recognized that her personal experience with heart disease was invaluable to her employer. Sarah knew that if she taught her staff about her experience, it would enrich their understanding and support her department's overall mission. And her heart problems would only make the issue of heart disease in women that much more personal and real. The more she thought about it, Sarah also recognized that her boss—who was also a nurse—would probably be pretty understanding, especially given Sarah's continued strong performance in her job.

So Sarah went ahead and told them. It took her a few weeks to get up the nerve, but she did it. At first her boss and the members of her staff were shocked and a bit put off that Sarah hadn't told them before. They'd all noticed that she was acting differently and they'd been gossiping, asking each other: What's the matter with Sarah? They'd been worried, so once they found out what had actually happened, it put them at ease— they were relieved. Sarah was relieved too, especially when her boss was supportive and kind. She found out that her staff still respects her and they really don't treat her any differently. They may occasionally ask how she's doing, but that's okay with Sarah. They encourage her and show compassion. One of Sarah's employees even told her that she seems more "real" now, "more human"—fallible, like everybody else. If you're concerned about whether or not to be open about your heart disease, consider Sarah's experience. Recognize that you'll feel more comfortable with everything out in the open and, although you can't control your coworkers' reactions, you can't predict them either.

Have a positive attitude. Some of the most surprising research on women and heart disease tells us that, when you return to work, your worries and fears can make you your own worst enemy. Your attitude about your own ability to do your job can make all the difference between whether you succeed or fail. In fact, one study showed that—regardless of your physical symptoms—if you think positively about your heart problems and your capabilities, you're far more likely to perform your work well.[4] How can you stop yourself from undermining your own success?

- *Know your limitations and capabilities.* Your doctor can give you clear guidance, encouragement, and support regarding your heart disease and your abilities. Talk to him or her about the specifics of your job and whether you'll have any problems performing that job, based on your heart condition.
- *Match your capabilities to your job.* If your doctor says you shouldn't have any problem standing on your feet six hours a day cutting hair, take her at her word. If she says you can sit at your desk for eight hours and handle routine office work, then assume that you're okay. If she says there's no reason you can't teach a classroom of second graders, then you should return to work with confidence.
- *Make your decisions based on reality.* Once you've made an accurate assessment of your abilities—with your doctor's help—and

---

4. Colleen Newvine, "Heart Disease, Work Performance, Mental Health All Connected," *The University Record Online*, http://www.umich.edu/~urecord/ 0405/ Dec13_04/09.shtml.

your job responsibilities, act accordingly. If your job matches your abilities, stop worrying. It will get in the way of your performance. Otherwise, take steps to find a job that better suits your condition.

- *Check your emotional health.* If your doctor's assessment of your abilities and your job description tells you everything's okay, but you're still experiencing anxiety or fear about performing your job, it may be an emotional issue. Get professional help if you need it (see Chapter 3).

Reinvent your job.   Maybe you need to reduce your hours in order to be able to comfortably do your job—at least, for a while. If your doctor says you're ready to go back to work, but you need to ease back a bit or you've decided that you'd be much happier working part time, don't be afraid to talk with your employer or supervisor. Many women are able to return to work on a part-time basis and gradually return to a full-time arrangement.

What if you want to turn your full-time job into a part-time one permanently? If you think that's your best long-term option and you can afford it, don't be afraid to make the switch. Here are a few tips on how to negotiate reduced hours or more job flexibility.

- *Do your homework.* Find out if there are other people in your company who have flexible or part-time jobs.
- *Develop a plan.* Analyze your job and determine which components you can keep and do effectively on a part-time basis.
- *Sell yourself.* Remind your supervisor of your record of strong performance—that you're a valuable and experienced contributor to the business. Provide reassurance that you will be fully capable of meeting your obligations.
- *Be sure to ask about health insurance.* Some companies do not offer benefits to part-time employees. Find out what your options are. Maybe you can arrange to prorate your benefits or pay a portion of your health insurance coverage.[5]

---

5. S. B. Dynerman and L. O. Hayes, *The Best Jobs in America for Parents* (New York: Rawson/Macmillan, 1991).

Know your rights.   If you're afraid of losing your job, remember: There are laws out there to protect you. Two federal statutes protect employees who are affected by illness: the Americans with Disabilities Act (ADA), and the Family and Medical Leave Act (FMLA).

- *The Americans with Disabilities Act* (ADA): The ADA protects you if you work for an employer who has fifteen or more employees and if you suffer a disability as defined by the statute. According to the statute, an individual with a disability is a person who has a physical or mental impairment that substantially limits one or more "major life activities," which includes activities such as caring for oneself, performing manual tasks, walking, seeing, hearing, speaking, breathing, learning, and working. Whether a person is disabled within the meaning of the statute is dependent on each individual's situation. This law prohibits employers from discriminating against qualified employees or prospective employees with disabilities in job application procedures, hiring, firing, advancement, compensation, job training, and other aspects of employment. A qualified employee or applicant with a disability is an individual who, with or without reasonable accommodation, can perform the essential functions of the job in question. If you need for your employer to provide certain accommodations so you can perform the essential functions of your job, the ADA requires the employer to work with you to come up with a reasonable accommodation. Examples of accommodations include: making existing facilities readily accessible and usable; job restructuring, modifying work schedules, reassignment to a vacant position; acquiring or modifying equipment; adjusting or modifying examinations, training materials, or policies; and providing qualified readers or interpreters. In very limited situations, employers may file for an "undue hardship" exception in cases where they believe making the accommodation would impose an undue hardship on the business. Undue hardship is defined as an action requiring significant difficulty or expense when considered in light of factors such as the size of the business, financial resources, and the nature and structure of its operations.

- *The Family and Medical Leave Act (FMLA).* Under the FMLA, if you need time off for treatment or surgery, or if you still suffer a serious health condition (as defined by the statute) at the time of your recovery and/or return to work, you may be eligible for twelve weeks of unpaid leave, which can be taken all at one time or intermittently. Keep in mind, if you're on unpaid leave, you may be eligible for short-term disability payments, if your employer provides those benefits. FMLA applies to all public agencies, including state, local, and federal employers, local education agencies (schools), and private-sector employers with fifty or more employees.

According to Angie Davis, an associate at the Memphis-based law firm of Baker, Donelson, Bearman, Caldwell & Berkowitz, PC, if you find that your employer is breaking either of these laws, here's what you can do:

1. Under the ADA, if you feel that your employer is not accommodating your disability or that you are being discriminated against because of your disability, you should first address your employer through the Human Resources Department.
2. If your employer doesn't cooperate, you can go to the Equal Employment Opportunity Commission (EEOC) to file a charge of discrimination. They will perform an investigation on your behalf.
3. The EEOC is a federal agency with offices throughout the United States. Office locations can be found at www.eeoc.gov.
4. The FMLA is not governed by this agency, so your only recourse under the FMLA is to file a lawsuit in federal court. This can be a very complicated process. You'll need to hire an attorney to represent you. If you believe you have grounds for such a suit and have trouble finding an affordable attorney, contact your local legal services agency for recommendations.

DEALING WITH COWORKERS

In earlier chapters, we talked about some of the ways in which your family relationships and friendships can change in the wake of a heart event.

Not surprisingly, relationships with coworkers can change as well. How your coworkers react to your illness can affect you emotionally—even leave you feeling isolated and alone.

You'll probably experience some of the same reactions at work that you've experienced at home and in your community. Some coworkers won't know what to say. They may feel awkward or embarrassed because they don't know you well enough to express their feelings or thoughts in an appropriate manner. Remember: Some people simply don't know how to be empathic or supportive when a fellow worker gets sick or injured. Like some of your friends and relatives, coworkers may find your illness frightening—they'll worry about you or they'll think about how it relates to something in their own life.

Those situations are not unique to the workplace, but this one is: Your boss or your colleagues may be concerned that you won't be able to keep up or do your work at the same pace you once did. It can cause resentment if they believe they'll have to pick up the slack due to your illness—and that's an issue you must address. If that happens, your best strategy is to educate your boss and/or your coworkers about your heart disease and your abilities—just as you educated your family. If your boss has questions, direct him or her to the WomenHeart Web site at www.womenheart.org or www.hearthealthywomen.org.

You might also consider doing a workshop at your office to educate the people you work with about heart disease. That can help reduce the stigma associated with being labeled a heart patient, give you a sense of control, minimize gossip, and alleviate some of the tension you might be experiencing. Guidance on how to raise awareness at work and develop an in-service educational program is available through the American Heart Association (see the Resources section).

MINIMIZE CONFLICTS TO REDUCE STRESS

No matter how much you endeavor to educate others, not every coworker will understand your situation. They may not empathize or care about what you've been through. Your illness may make you more vulnerable to a difficult coworker. To reduce work-related stress, you'll want to minimize conflicts with fellow coworkers. Here are some tips:

Be empathic.   Use empathy instead of anger in responding. Maybe your coworker has a long history of tough times and just can't cope with another person having a problem. Using empathy will diffuse your frustrations and reduce the chances of having a distressing confrontation. Remember it's likely that the problem is with your fellow coworker, not you.

Turn the tables.   You may want to try befriending this person. Ask her, "How are you doing?" or "How's your life?" Be genuine. Kindness works wonders to defuse situations.

Practice avoidance.   Sometimes you have to know when it's time to walk away and ignore a conflict. Recognize that some people enjoy conflict, live with it every day, and gain power from the energy. Frequently these types of people gain more power when you respond by getting angry. So just ignore them and move on.

Use conflict-resolution techniques.   If the coworker continues to badger you or continuously tries to engage you in a fight, back off. Then use the conflict-resolution techniques discussed in Chapter 6 on pages 117.

Seek help from the authorities.   If a conflict is interfering with your ability to do your job, seek help from your supervisor or your Human Relations Department. Be prepared: Do your homework and be ready to provide details about the specific issue that created the problem. Focus only on the facts. Provide paperwork if it's available. Avoid emotionalism; it gets you nowhere. Don't personalize what this coworker says or does to you. Remember: In all likelihood, if this coworker has acted this way with you, he/she has done it to others.

Unbearable situations.   Sometimes heart patients find that their coworkers have such difficulty dealing with their illness that they decide to make a change.

> *At the time of my heart attack, I was a program manager with six men working under my direction. I went back to work six weeks after my heart attack and started working just a few hours each day. I was in shock when I returned to work. People who I'd thought I had a close working relationship with all of a sudden*

would duck into bathrooms, cubicles, or turn the other way when they saw me coming. Others would stare at my chest and say, "You don't look like you had a heart attack." My own team of men turned into a bunch of mother hens, with the exception of one who told me that he couldn't really talk or look at me because it reminded him of his father's death from a heart attack. The other five men would try very hard to keep me from getting involved in any stressful developments, so much so that I eventually didn't even know what was going on with my own company. My supervisor, who had previously assigned the most challenging tasks to my group, now became patronizing and cruel to me. When he'd give me an assignment, he'd usually finish by saying, "Now, you're not going to drop dead from doing this, are you? It wouldn't look good for business."

—Tasha, Hot Springs, AR, age 40

Tasha's experience is not as unusual as you might imagine. Women report a mix of reactions from coworkers, including avoidance, curiosity, overprotectiveness, and downright cruelty. Obviously, it's difficult to do your job under such conditions. Tasha's work environment had become a place that was no longer safe emotionally. After several months, her doctor told her to make a decision: "Today is the day you must choose what you want," he said. "Every day you work in that environment, you're putting yourself under tremendous stress by trying to ignore what your coworkers are doing and working with people who don't root for you. You're shortening your life." Tasha never went back to work that day. In fact, that was Tasha's last day at that job. She made a choice that many women with heart disease have to make. At the age of forty, she left her job after working there for twenty years.

CHANGING JOBS

When my kids were young, and long before my heart troubles began, I wanted to leave my job as a hospital-based social worker because it was too demanding. The work hours weren't clearly defined, the stress was tremendous, and there were emergencies on a daily basis.

As a first step, I drew up a list of what I wanted and my goals. I wanted to see my children more than on weekends. I knew I wanted to work closer to my home. I wanted more flexible hours. I wanted to expand my skills. I wanted to make more money for the time I put in on the job.

Then I formulated a job-hunting plan. I began talking to people, looking in the paper, and making phone calls to professionals I had previously networked with. I talked to friends and family to find leads. I looked in the phone book and made a list of names of people I might want to work with. I made phone calls. I became a woman with a mission and a drive to improve my work life.

By taking those steps and knowing my goals and dreams, I found a wonderful job in private practice that literally changed my life and greatly reduced my stress level. If you're ready to change jobs, defining your needs and your dreams is the best place to start. Then the hunt begins.

Make a wish list.   First think about some preferred traits you want in a job. Ask yourself the following questions and write down your answers:

1.   Would it help you to have a job where you worked more defined hours?
2.   Would it help you to work closer to home, the grocery store, and your children's school?
3.   Do you want a job where you can actually have time to eat lunch and relax during a portion of your workday?
4.   Do you need a job that is flexible with the demands on your life outside of work?
5.   Do you have enough time to exercise during your workday?
6.   Is your job creative enough and challenging enough to motivate you and keep you interested?

Incorporate all those answers into a list of traits you want from your next job. Let that list be your guide.

Use a career counselor.   If you're stuck, a career counselor can help you sort through the possibilities and get you on the right track. You can find career counselors at nearby universities or colleges or you can visit the National Career Development Association (see the Resources section) for guidance on how to find one in your area. The NCDA Web site offers comprehensive listings of career counselors and centers all over the country by state and city.

Start networking.   Talk to everyone you know and create a web of contacts. In *The 2006 What Color Is Your Parachute?*, here's what author Richard Nelson Bolles recommends:

- Talk to family, friends, and your community networks about possible job openings or opportunities.
- Go directly to a place of business that interests you, whether they have an opening or not. Ask about opportunities. Tell them exactly what position you're interested in and why you're right for it.
- Look for businesses in the Yellow Pages that fall within your area of interest and expertise. Then call them and ask about the kind of jobs you're looking for and how to pursue them.

LANDING THE JOB

Once you've uncovered an opportunity, it's time to sell yourself. As a heart patient, you'll be walking into an interview with a unique set of concerns. Approach a job interview with a positive attitude—but recognize that discrimination can happen. Having heart disease simply compounds the potential problems. Because you have a preexisting medical condition, employers may be concerned about the possibility of increased insurance premiums and other added, long-range costs. That's especially true if you're overweight and have heart disease. It's not unusual for employers to have preconceived notions about people who are overweight, associating it with laziness and lack of motivation. And age discrimination can happen too. Of course, it's illegal to discriminate against someone on the basis of their age or weight, but such cases are not always easy to prove. Better to use your initiative on the front end to counter those assumptions. How?

- *It's your job to sell yourself.* Your mission is to obliterate any employer's preconceived notions about you.

- *Research the position.* Know what the job involves, including the responsibilities and what your employer will expect from you.
- *Tell the employer how your skills and talents match their needs.* Tell them everything you can about your experience and abilities. Let them know that you're proud of the depth of your experience and that it will only enhance your job performance, effectiveness, and productivity.
- *Be confident, poised and energetic.* Go in trusting yourself and your abilities, and project a positive attitude and image. That will go a long way toward making a good impression and countering any preconceptions about your age or health.
- *Remember: How you look is very important.* Wear fresh, professional, contemporary clothes that you feel comfortable in. Have a fashion show! Try on your job interview outfit for a friend or your partner a few days in advance and get a second opinion. That will help boost your confidence.

DEALING WITH HEALTH ISSUES DURING YOUR INTERVIEW

As you approach a job interview, you'll probably be concerned about whether your illness will affect your chances of getting a job. Can they ask questions about your health? What should you tell them about your heart condition?

Know your rights.   First of all, it's important for you to know that, under the Americans with Disabilities Act, it's illegal for an employer to ask questions about your health unless they've made a conditional job offer. In other words, during your initial interview, it's illegal for an interviewer to ask questions such as, "Do you have any health problems?" or, "Have you ever had any health problems?" Still, you're not going to want to confront an interviewer if he or she raises such questions. Instead, immediately following the interview, write the discussion down so you'll have a record of it, no matter what happens.

What if they ask anyway.   "How is your health?" or "How much were you absent from your last job?" or even "I see you've been on leave for two months, why is that?" Remember, they are looking for reassurance, not details. Respond honestly, but don't give them more information than they need. You might say: "I have heart disease, but it won't have any affect on my ability to do the job. My productivity, compared to other workers, is excellent." Or "I missed some work at my last job because I was sick. I discovered that I have heart disease, but it's under control and I am on medication for it. I don't expect it to interfere in any way with my ability to do my job—and that includes my ability to be at work every day." If the employer doesn't make you a job offer, and you suspect this was because of your age or health status, you should report it to the Equal Employment Opportunity Commission (see the Resources section) and file a charge. Again, be sure to write the content of the interview down.

Don't volunteer any extra information. Given that it's illegal, an interviewer will probably not ask you directly about your health. Instead, he or she may ask a question that might lead you to talk about your health, or make a provocative comment about illness, exercise, diet, or leaves of

> When I interviewed for my job I didn't tell the director about my heart problem, because I didn't want it to factor in one way or the other. My heart would not be the reason I couldn't do the job. I told them several months later when we were at a staff retreat in Yosemite, and I chose not to do the climb of Half Dome. They knew I was an athlete and wondered why I wasn't up to the challenge, but completely understood once they all knew. Since they already knew me and knew that I could do my job well, they didn't judge me because I had a heart problem.
> —Margaret, Fresno, CA, age 36

You are under no obligation to reveal information about your heart condition during an initial interview. In fact, unless it comes up or relates directly to the job itself, you won't want to discuss your heart condition before you take the job. However, once you start working, it's wise to tell your boss and your coworkers about your heart disease as soon as possible—for your own safety. If you have a heart attack at work or a health-related issue arises, your coworkers will know what to do. They won't be caught off guard—and you won't be caught without the support you need.

absence followed by a pause. Resist filling in the blank. Don't volunteer health-related information that you haven't been asked about. You are under no legal obligation to tell them about your health. But don't be evasive. If the subject comes up, be straightforward and direct.

Practice positive responses.   It's important to be honest, but just as important to focus on your strengths. Be clear that you are fully capable and willing to do the job, and that you'll do it as well if not better than any of their other employees. Exuding confidence and determination in the face of heart disease only makes you look stronger

A conditional offer.   Sometimes employers make a job offer that's conditional upon a medical examination, drug test, or some other evaluation. In such cases, you may be asked to go through a medical exam. At that point, an employer can legally ask questions about your health or disability. And once the evaluation process is complete, the employer can eliminate you from consideration for the job based on your health. However, they must be able to prove that your disability will interfere with your ability to do the job, even if they take steps to accommodate your needs. If this happens to you and you feel you've been treated unfairly, again, visit the EEOC Web site and decide if you want to file a charge.

Find out more.   States and municipalities have their own rules and regulations about what can be asked during a job interview. If you're concerned about it, do some research on your state and local laws. You can generally find this information through your state or local labor department; by searching the Internet for "worker's rights" and your state name; or by consulting with your local librarian—he or she can direct you to the right resources.

The U.S. Equal Employment Opportunity Commission and the U.S. Department of Labor offer additional information concerning your rights under the Americans with Disabilities Act. Follow the links below for further information:

- www.eeoc.gov/policy/docs/preemp.html
- www.dol.gov/odep/archives/ek96/inquiry.htm

Health-insurance Issues

As a heart patient, it's particularly important that you maintain insurance coverage when you change jobs. Here are some general guidelines to make sure your insurance continues uninterrupted:

1. *If you are changing jobs or insurers, be sure that you do not have a break between insurance plans for more than sixty-two days.* The Health Insurance Portability and Accountability Act (HIPAA) limits the extent to which some group health plans can exclude coverage for preexisting conditions. In order to continue your health insurance, you need to make sure you've had health insurance that's considered "creditable"—that is, health-insurance coverage for at least twelve months without a break of more than sixty-two days. If you meet those conditions when you change jobs and you send the new insurance company the HIPAA Creditable Coverage notice from your previous health plan, the new insurance plan cannot refuse to cover your preexisting conditions.

2. *If you are about to change jobs or lose your health coverage, ask your employer about COBRA coverage before you make the change.* COBRA (Consolidated Omnibus Budget Reconciliation Act of 1985) is another federal law that protects you and helps you to buy benefits when you are between jobs. When you change jobs, there's usually a probationary period before your health insurance kicks in and you'll need COBRA coverage to bridge the time gap. You must be proactive in getting this coverage, even though your current employer is required to inform you about COBRA. Under federal COBRA, you become responsible for the total cost of your health-insurance coverage plus a 2 percent administration fee. But it allows you to stay insured and it may enable you to wait out the gap period until you become covered under the health plan at your new job. The maximum amount of time that you can extend your coverage under COBRA is usually eighteen months or until you get coverage under another group health plan without pre-existing condition limitations.

3. *Be proactive and talk with your current health administrator about COBRA continuation if you are changing jobs.* Under COBRA law, if you leave your job the employer is required to notify you of your COBRA rights within fourteen to forty-four days after the date your coverage under their health plan coverage is terminated. You then have sixty days to enroll in COBRA and another forty-five days to pay the premiums. However, the employer is only required to mail you the COBRA notice; the employer is not required to make sure you actually received the notice. If the COBRA notice is mailed to you but is lost or stolen in the mail, you could lose your opportunity to enroll in COBRA. To avoid loss of coverage and preexisting condition limitations, make sure that you enroll in COBRA within thirty days of the date you change jobs. Again, it is up to you to be on top of the process and to make sure that all of the paperwork is done and received in a timely manner for you to receive COBRA.

4. *If you're changing jobs, seek out an employer with a good health-insurance program.* Large corporations, hospitals and universities are more likely to offer strong benefits than are small businesses. The bigger the employer, the more likely it is to offer health insurance to part-time employees. When you're job hunting, be creative. Seek out employers who are more likely to offer outstanding health-insurance coverage.

5. *Find out more.* For more information on HIPAA, COBRA or other short-term insurance solutions visit:

    -   www.quotit.net/resources/terms_health2.htm
    -   info.insure.com/health/hipaa.html
    -   www.dol.gov/dol/topic/health-plans/portability.htm
    -   www.dol.gov/dol/topic/health-plans/cobra.htm

SOME WOMEN CHOOSE EARLY RETIREMENT

If you've been in the workforce for a long time, you may have reached the point where you look at work and life differently. If you can afford to stop working in the wake of a heart event, you may well be ready to do so. You're likely to know exactly what you want to do with your time and energy. You're also likely to have a more secure grasp of what the possibilities are for you than you did when you were younger. Your goals, your aspirations, your priorities, and perspective have probably shifted. Maybe you want to spend more time traveling, taking classes, and indulging your hobbies. In all likelihood, your goals no longer revolve around work. Your brush with heart disease may well have intensified your desire to branch out, expand your horizons, and embrace what author Gail Sheehy calls your Second Adulthood. Just think of all of the paths you can take.

> *Most women come to realize that they have been defined in their First Adulthood by their relation to others—the parents, husbands, children, bosses, and mentors for whom they performed. Now is the time to construct one's own new Second Adulthood identity.*
> —Gail Sheehy, *Sex and the Seasoned Woman*, 2006

Some women in their second adulthood can finally do things they could never do before, so they cherish their new freedom and sense of self. They have their own choices for filling their time and they enjoy each moment exploring their options.

> *I never looked back after leaving my job as president of a steel supply company that I had started. That was a job I truly loved. But I became involved with my children's school functions (I'm not sure how much they really liked this). I became a band mom and volunteered every chance I got. It made me feel so fulfilled and kept my mind on other things. I thought less and less about my physical woes. My mind was in overdrive most of the time, and I thought of ways to keep active and alert. For the first time, I attempted needlepoint and was amazed at how well I could do it. I became addicted and then added cross-stitching, and made a Mother Goose quilt. I tried oil painting and painted small laughing clowns and handed them out as gifts. Some people thought I was not taking my health seriously and was in denial. I took my health seriously by not dwelling on my problems day in and day out. I knew my limitations but I just wanted to truly live each day to the fullest with the spirit, mind, and body that I was still blessed with!*
> —Mary Rose, Houston, TX, age 62

WHAT IF YOU HAVE TO STOP WORKING?

For some women, the problems associated with heart disease can become so severe that it's necessary to stop working. In most cases this isn't something that happens overnight. In fact, it can be a long and arduous process. But at some point it becomes clear that working full time is no longer an option. If this occurs, your doctor will be actively involved in the decision. For the sake of your health, he or she will advise you to leave your job.

> *Emotionally you're never really ready to say that you're "disabled." But I look at it this way, what choice did I really have? Being described by the government as "disabled" doesn't mean your life is over—it doesn't define who you are or what you're capable of. Moving beyond this hurdle takes time. Doctors don't want you to bear this label either—they're worried about its impact on you emotionally, socially, and physically. But eventually the reality hit all of us: I could no longer do things at work the same way I always had. I was the person who ran things. I was the doer, the problem solver, the organizer—and over time I knew I couldn't physically do all of it at the same level. After two bypasses, I had to start thinking about myself—my health and my life. To get another job—one that involved less stress and fewer responsibilities, I knew I'd have to dumb down my resume or I would be overqualified. That option was totally unappealing and impractical. And I wouldn't know how to do that anyway. Scaling down and accepting my heart problems is okay. As for receiving disability payments, it doesn't bother me. After all, I'm entitled to these benefits; I've paid for them!*
>
> —Lucy, New York, NY, age 59

Sometimes your heart disease leaves you no choice. If it becomes problematic and stressful to work at the level and capacity that you're accustomed to, it's time to assess your overall well-being with your doctor. If, because of your medical limitations, working in your job—or any job—will cause you further suffering, your doctor(s) can document that information in your records. While your doctor can evaluate you medically, it's important for you to be totally honest and open about how you're feeling so she can accurately assess your situation. If your doctor(s) conclude that you're no longer able to work, you may become eligible for Social Security Disability Insurance (SSDI) and/or Supplemental Security Income (SSI). Applying to either SSDI, SSI, or even private disability insurance is a process. It will take time and it's quite cumbersome—so be prepared for that.

Disability payments provide a stream of regular monthly income, but most heart patients report a substantial change in their lives—financially, socially, and emotionally. The women quoted here—Billie, Lucy, and Tasha—each made major adjustments to her lifestyle and self-image when she qualified for disability, but all emerged with a strong sense of gratitude and a positive outlook.

> *I'm deemed permanently disabled due to the severity of my heart condition. During 2001, my heart disease made me quite ill, and it was a constant source of stress and anxiety to keep my condition under wraps. I was in middle management—and even with my heart troubles I was able to continue to do my job well. I basically ran the show throughout my career and for my staff of twenty-five in an international investment-banking firm. There wasn't too much scrutiny, until I started having to be hospitalized for three to four weeks at a time. We have suffered much since that time, financially, emotionally, and physically. What's truly important is the very real fact that I'm still here in spite of it all ... even with CHF [congestive heart failure] stage IV.*
>
> —Billie, Las Vegas, NV, age 44

Given Billie's high-powered job in the financial sector, she and her family had a great deal of financial freedom. Once she went on disability, Billie's income dropped substantially. It changed their lives. Billie's daughter had been attending an expensive private school that they could no longer afford. She not only had to switch schools, but also had to change her plans for college due to the family's new financial constraints. It's not uncommon for a woman's disability to affect the entire family and generate acute feelings of loss. That can be hard on everyone. I encourage you to refer back to Chapter 2 (The Stages of Grief) for a discussion of grappling with loss, and Chapter 6 (Coping with Change: Your Family) for insights into how your family might regain its balance.

After leaving her job at the investment bank, Billie has tried to find work that would match her skills and her limitations as a heart patient—but that's difficult to do and can be quite frustrating. Even though she's receiving payments through Social Security Disability Insurance (SSDI), Billie can still work. However, her monthly income must remain below a certain level every month—and that level is well below what she used to earn. So Billie's situation is not unlike Lucy's; she would be hopelessly overqualified for a job that pays the salary she's eligible to receive. Once you qualify for SSDI, the amount of money you can earn each year is limited. For further information, visit www.ssa.gov or check with your local Social Security office.

For most women, the emotional issues match the financial repercussions of going on disability insurance. Being told that you are permanently disabled can be very difficult to handle, adding to feelings of helplessness and hopelessness that come with heart disease.

> *I was the main bread winner in the family and when I stopped working, I felt like damaged goods—first in my role as a wife and mother and, then, as an unemployed member of society. Suddenly, I needed other people's help in every area of my life and that's something I wasn't used to. It hasn't been easy,*
>
> —Tasha, Hot Springs, AR, age 40

How have women like Lucy, Billie, and Tasha managed to move forward? Here are a few things all three have in common:

- They have a positive attitude. They're grateful that they've survived and have the ability to appreciate all of life's gifts.
- They're relieved to have social security disability payments coming in every month. All of these women look at SSDI as a program that they've paid into, so they feel perfectly comfortable accepting these payments because they need it—they've earned it.
- They no longer let the stigma of being disabled get them down. They've had to work hard to process their feelings about being disabled and turn their thinking around. If you're having trouble

accepting the fact that you have to be on disability, don't hesitate to seek counseling. This is a new reality and requires a major adjustment. (See Chapter 3, Getting the Help You Need.)

- All three spend their time volunteering, which fills their lives with meaning and usefulness.

- They feel that, for the first time in their lives, their time is their own. They choose what they'll spend their time doing every day based on how they're feeling. They have time to rest and to be with their grandchildren and children. An enormous amount of stress has gone out of their lives—and an enormous amount of joy has come in!

SOCIAL SECURITY DISABILITY INSURANCE AND SUPPLEMENTAL SECURITY INCOME: THE BASICS

Social Security Disability Insurance (SSDI).

- When you work and pay Social Security taxes you earn Social Security credits that can qualify you for disability insurance—this applies to the self-employed as well as those who've worked for an employer. You've also been earning Medicare protection while you worked.

- If you worked long enough to qualify, you may be eligible for disability benefits under Social Security. Your doctor will determine if you are disabled—that is, unable to work at your previous job or any other job because of your medical condition(s). To qualify, your disability must be severe enough that it will last at least a year or could result in your death.

- Your Social Security benefits will represent a percentage of your average lifetime earnings. A worker with average earnings can expect to replace about 40 percent of his or her average lifetime earnings. If you check the statement you receive annually from the Social Security Administration, it will give you an idea of what your benefits will be. Or go to www.ssa.gov, where you'll find a calculator for figuring out your benefits.

- Social Security is intended to supplement other income sources through your pensions, savings or investments, and insurance plans.
- It can take several months for Social Security to process your claim. So don't delay. Visit your local Social Security office as soon as you can to file.
- In some cases, you are allowed to work but for a minimal amount of time and money. Check with your Social Security office.

Supplemental Security Income (SSI). These are disability payments for people who have few resources or low income. The amount of income you receive will be based on your income, resources and where you live. The federal government typically pays a basic amount and then the state you live in adds money to that. If you are eligible for SSI, you are likely to be eligible for other assistance from the state, such as food stamps and Medicaid.

Unlike SSDI, SSI is not based on your work history. The payments of SSI come from general tax revenues, not through Social Security taxes.

How to Apply. To apply for either SSDI or SSI you will need your birth certificate, a marriage certificate (if your spouse is applying) and your most recent W-2 form (or tax return if you are self-employed).

ADVICE FROM HEART PATIENTS REGARDING SSDI

- Don't be too disappointed if you get turned down for SSDI. It happens frequently. Appeal the decision and reapply. Don't give up.
- Hire a lawyer or financial planner to help guide you through the process.
- Get as many doctors as possible to confirm that you're disabled. There is power in having multiple doctors support each other's opinions.
- Be aware this is a complicated pain-in-the-neck process with a ton of paperwork. Just be assertive and patient. It will happen. Remember Social Security is a bureaucracy.

For more information about either SSDI or SSI, visit www.socialsecurity.gov or call toll free 1-800-772-1213.

HEALTH-INSURANCE COVERAGE AND DISABILITY

Fortunately, I had a benefits plan from my employer that paid my insurance and me for the first six months after my last day of my work. It took me seven months to become approved for disability, so there was only a lapse of one month on my income. But health insurance was a whole new nightmare. Our government system is quirky if you ask me. When a person becomes permanently disabled, their disability checks start immediately but they don't qualify for Medicare for TWO years! So for those two years I had to pay the COBRA price for my health insurance, which was $900 a month. Had I not had a husband to help with this, I would have just had to let my health care and medications slide for those two years.

—Tasha, Hot Springs, AR, age 40

When you first stop working, COBRA coverage may be your only insurance option (see pages 175–176). So be sure to talk to your health-insurance administrator about COBRA before you leave your job.

ONWARD AND UPWARD

Doubtless you've already had plenty of experience dealing with the health-care system. In Chapter 9, we'll explore the best ways to approach insurers, doctors, and health-care facilities, including strategies for communicating more effectively. This is where you'll find out more about how to become your own best health-care advocate.

chapter nine

NEGOTIATING THE
HEALTH-CARE SYSTEM

Home Alone—Nothing seems to happen during the day. One night she sits up and says her heart is skipping. She feels bloated and can't breathe. Her abdomen looks like a starving child's— she's got a very large belly. We were told to cut down on salt. Cut down? No one told us from what level to what level, so I was feeding her chicken broth like the book said. I gave her heart-healthy food. I was trying to do the right thing by changing her diet. In reality, I was feeding her way too much salt and causing fluid buildup around her heart and lungs.

What this is about is being given minimal information at the wrong time. It took us nearly a year to educate ourselves in what, I guess, doctors and nurses consider common knowledge. Actually, we should have received this information as the first wave of support after leaving the hospital. I wonder how much money is wasted on return hospital visits due to a lack of accurate educational information being given to patients and their families at a time when they're actually capable of processing it.

—Tina's husband Billy, Vaughan, MS, age 62

Billy has faced what so many caregivers and patients do when trying to negotiate a medical system that doesn't always cater to the needs of its consumers. Sometimes it seems as if the entire health-care system runs on autopilot—and that it's not tuned in to the emotional and educational needs of patients and their families. Typically, patients and their families are inundated with paper—pamphlets, brochures, and articles from the doctor's office or hospital. Unfortunately, these educational tools don't have the impact that comes with direct face-to-face communication with health-care providers. Plus the timing can be a problem. All too often patients and their families receive educational information and instructions in the midst of a medical crisis, when they're less likely to be able to focus on it or remember it later. Then, once they've left the hospital and are craving information, they don't have a clue who to ask or what to ask for. That's one of the reasons a timely follow-up with your health-care provider after your heart event is so important.

To further complicate matters, most patients and their families don't understand medical terms, which makes it even harder for them to be well informed. The lack of attention to detail associated with meeting the needs of patients and their families can cause undue stress and anxiety. And that's due, in part, to dramatic changes in the health-care system during the past few decades. There is no doubt that patients in the United States have better access to improved medications, medical treatments, and diagnostic tools than they did many years ago, but the patient and doctor relationship has become a more complex and difficult one.

> *Medical knowledge has rapidly expanded in recent years, but medical care has in certain crucial ways deteriorated. For a whole complex of reasons, doctors and patients eye each other with mistrust.*
> —Edward Shorter, Doctors and Their Patients[1]

Yes, medicine has changed. Office visits to your doctor used to be more relaxed and less rushed. It seemed as if you had more face-to-face time with your doctor. Not only did you receive a thorough examination, but also there was time to talk—and not just about medical issues. Questions were asked and answered, and there was the added luxury of being able to ask a question again if necessary.[2] Remember when doctors would

---

1. Edward Shorter, *Doctors and Their Patients* (Piscataway, NJ: Transaction Publisher, 1991).

2. F. Davidoff, MD, "Time," *Annals of Internal Medicine* 127 (6) (1997): 483–85.

actually visit you at home? Maybe you don't. Like dinosaurs, house calls are virtually extinct. When I was a girl, the doctor would come by the house when I was sick—he'd visit, listen, examine, prescribe, counsel, and, most of all, reassure everyone. In some ways, your doctor was like a part of the family. Ah . . . the good ole days!

In his book, *Building Patient/Doctor Trust,* Dr. Frank Boehm zeros in on what he considers a critical issue for patients and doctors—the importance of establishing trust. Dr. Boehm believes that when patients and doctors have a strained relationship, it affects the patient's overall health outcome, creates frustration, and can lead to lawsuits. [3] A 2004 Harris Poll has shown that patients were more concerned about whether their doctor had good interpersonal skills than about his or her training and knowledge of new medical treatments. What these patients wanted was a doctor who didn't make them wait too long; a doctor who spent time with them, listened to them, was easy to talk to, took their concerns seriously, and showed care and respect.[4] Patients, it seems, are starved for a positive interpersonal connection with their doctors.

What's getting in the way of the patient/doctor connection? It's the need for medical efficiency and cost-effectiveness, and the nature of health-insurance reimbursements. There is no question that doctors want to help their patients through careful and professional diagnoses and treatment. But nowadays doctors are worried about all of the paperwork they have to do to be reimbursed by insurers. That takes time and energy, and is incredibly cumbersome. They also face rising concerns about liability issues—given the increased threat of lawsuits and the rising cost of liability insurance. All these issues have an impact on the patient/doctor relationship.

Today the focus of medicine tends to be on patients in crisis rather than on prevention, an approach that could keep more people from getting sick in the first place.

One study showed that less than half the time doctors spend with high-risk patients is spent talking about risk-factor reduction, such as

---

3. Frank Boehm, *Building Doctor/Patient Trust* (self-published, 2006).

4. News Release regarding *Wall Street Journal Online,* Harris Interactive Health-Care Poll, "Doctors' Interpersonal Skills Valued More Than Their Training or Being Up-to-Date," October 1, 2004, http://www.harrisinteractive.com/news/allnewsbydate.asp?NewsID=850.

diet and exercise. According to the study, the medical system has failed to put enough emphasis on training doctors to counsel patients about prevention. In addition, doctors have less incentive to practice preventive medicine, because they receive a lower reimbursement from insurers for time spent on prevention compared to time spent on diagnosis and treatment.[5] They're just not paid as much to help people stay healthy!

To make things worse, the health-care system is simply not user friendly. In fact, sometimes, it's just as difficult for doctors to negotiate the health-care system as it is for patients. Health-care plans don't place any value on warm, personal contact. In order to survive, doctors are forced to sacrifice quality time with patients. They have to spend more time on paperwork and administrative tasks than ever before.

Many doctors had rose-colored glasses on when they went through medical school, residency, and fellowships. Doubtless they had good intentions—they imagined their medical practices would be something like life on the popular television series of the 1970s, *Marcus Welby, M.D.* But once they'd gone through the rigorous training and years of experience, they found themselves working in an environment that wasn't made for the Dr. Welbys of the world.

In reality, physicians spend an average of sixteen minutes per visit with each patient.[6] It's no wonder preventive strategies aren't likely to be discussed. And with these time constraints, you can imagine how difficult it is for patients and their family members to become informed consumers. How is it possible to accurately understand and process the information you're given in a brief, sixteen-minute visit? How can you get all the details you need to make informed decisions about diagnostic interventions and treatments? What about understanding the medicines you're taking? And when will you be able to ask questions?

In order to begin to answer some of these questions, you first need to know your rights as a patient. In 1997, President Bill Clinton appointed a

---

5. J. Ma, G. G. Urizar, T. Alehegn, and R. S. Stafford, "Diet and Physical Activity Counseling During Ambulatory Care Visits in the United States," *Preventive Medicine* 39 (2004): 815–22.

6. E. Hing, D. K. Cherry, D. A. Woodwell, et al., National Ambulatory Medical Survey: 2004 Summary, Advance Data from Vital and Health Statistics, U.S. Department of Health and Human Services, Centers for Disease Control and Prevention, National Center for Health Statistics, June 2006: 374.

commission[7] to create guidelines for protecting and ensuring patients' rights. By 1998, the commission had issued a Consumer Bill of Rights and Responsibilities for the health-care industry. Although the bill didn't pass, its guiding principles have since been adopted by many U.S. health-care plans, including federally sponsored plans. These are principles that you should know, embrace, use, and expect in practice from your health-care provider, health-care plan, and health-care facility. Ideally, understanding these rights will empower you to be your own best health-care advocate and consumer.

YOUR PATIENT BILL OF RIGHTS

- *Information disclosure.* Patients can only make informed decisions about their health care, health plan, or health providers if the information is given to them in an understandable way. Health-care providers and facilities must make every effort to accommodate you if you have a mental and/or physical disability, language barrier, or just don't understand the information. You also have the right to have your questions answered in a timely fashion. Importantly, you have the right to choose not to participate in research studies, even IF your doctor asks you to participate; and that choice should not change the doctor/patient relationship.
- *A choice of providers and plans.* To gain access to appropriate and high-quality health care, you have the right to appropriate options in choosing your health-care providers. In addition, you have the right to know all of the credentials and names of all of the providers that are involved in your care and treatment.
- *Access to emergency services.* If you need emergency health care, you have the right to go to the emergency room of your choice, when you need it, to receive appropriate medical services without prior authorization or fear of financial penalty.
- *Participation in treatment decisions.* You have the right to actively participate in your health-care decisions about your care and

---

7. Advisory Commission on Consumer Protection and Quality in the Health Care Industry, appointed March 26, 1997, by President Bill Clinton.

treatment. If you can't participate in this process, other designated family members, guardians, or individuals can be appointed to do so. You have the right to put legal directives in
place, so that the medical team that takes care of you honors
your wishes.

- *Respect and nondiscrimination.* You have the right to have health-
care providers and health-plan representatives who treat you
with respect, are considerate of you, and are nondiscriminatory
in providing your care.
- *Confidentiality of health information.* You have the right to have
your confidentiality and your health-care information protected
by your health-care providers and health-care plan. You have the
right to have access to and copy all of your medical records. You
also have the right to ask your doctor to change your medical
records, if you find that they contain information that's irrele-
vant, inaccurate, or incomplete.
- *Complaints and Appeals*—You have the right to a timely and fair
process of reviewing complaints whether it concerns your
health-care providers, health-care plans, or hospitals. These
complaints can range from the conduct of certain personnel to
the adequacy of the health-care facility treating you.

YOUR RESPONSIBILITIES AS A PATIENT

- Actively participate in your own health-care decisions.
- Do what you can do to maximize your health by making healthy
lifestyle choices.
- Work in partnership with your health-care team in following
through with the treatment plan.
- Be honest and open in communicating your needs and wants to
your medical team.
- Be respectful and considerate of your health-care team.
- Understand that health professionals are not gods and medicine
is not a perfect science.
- Recognize that health-care professionals take care of many pa-
tients and are as efficient and fair as possible.
- Consciously try not to spread disease.

- Make a real effort to fulfill your financial obligations.
- Learn as much as you can about your health-care plans or health-care plan options. Become educated about what your plan covers and what it doesn't. Be your own best health-care consumer. Be prepared, so there will be fewer surprises.
- Know and follow your health-care plan's policies and procedures.
- Address your concerns about your health plan through the proper internal channels and appeals process.
- Be a conscientious health consumer. If you suspect that there's something illegal happening with your health-care plan, providers, or health-care facilities, report it to the proper authorities.

For more information about your rights and responsibilities as a patient visit http://www.hcqualitycommission.gov/final/append_a.html or http://www.consumer.gov/qualityhealth/rights.htm.

While knowing these rights and responsibilities empowers patients to take charge of their own health care, they obviously need to partner with their health-care providers to get the best quality health care available. What can you do to be an effective partner with your health-care providers?

WHAT'S UP DOC? YOU'VE GOT THE POWER

For the most part, medical professionals are wonderful, but keep in mind that they are not God. They are human just like you. You deserve to be treated with respect and if you are not satisfied with your diagnosis, treatment options, or even the respect given to you, then shop around until you find a doctor who will help you plan your future of living—and living well. Don't settle for any less.

—Tasha, Hot Springs, AR, age 40

Getting a doctor who's a good fit isn't always as easy as it sounds. Like so many relationships, it's a partnership. That means it depends on good communication and a certain amount of comfort and ease. Those are the keys to a good doctor/patient relationship, which is, in turn, the key to getting the medical care you need. If you find that the relationship makes you uncomfortable and the communication is problematic, it might be a good time to change doctors.

*The cardiology group I saw following my heart attack did not an-
swer my questions. I rarely saw the same cardiologist. I saw the
nurse practitioner more than the doctors. Their system of care
made me uncomfortable. So I asked the nurses at my cardiac rehabilitation for some recommendations. They suggested the doctor I
have now. She always has time for my questions.*

—Ashley, Phoenix, AZ, age 48

Don't assume that, because a doctor is brilliant and well respected, he or she is necessarily the right physician for you. Every patient is unique—and you may have very specific needs. Be patient. It may take a good bit of your time and energy to find the doctor who's right for you, but it's worth the effort. In fact, the relationship you develop with your physician can make an enormous difference in your overall health and well-being, so take the time to investigate your options and ask questions.

How Do You Go About Looking for a Doctor?

- Get referrals and network with your friends, family, and work colleagues to find out who they'd recommend.
- If you're lucky enough to know some doctors through work, volunteering, or your community, talk to them. Ask for their opinion and recommendations.
- Get on the Internet and Google the prospective doctor's name—look for any research articles or studies that the doctor's written or been an investigator for.
- If possible, review his/her training and education background, and read any other articles about the doctor that may be pertinent to your selection process. Sometimes local magazines run stories about the best doctors in the community.
- As you go through this process, you might see a pattern of names that rise to the top of your list. Those are the doctors you'll want to find out more about or interview.

Sometimes it's hard to know exactly what qualities you're looking for in a physician. For instance, if you've been referred to a top surgeon

BECOMING YOUR OWN BEST HEALTH ADVOCATE:
HOW TO WORK WITH YOUR DOCTORS
AND THE MEDICAL COMMUNITY

Women can make a difference in their medical care and reduce their risk for heart disease by making positive lifestyle changes and taking medications that help them control their risk factors.

In preparation for a visit to your doctor's office, it's important that you be proactive. Keep a log of your major complaints and, before your visit, make a list of three to six questions. That gives you a lot of power. It's important for you to talk to your doctor to find out how you can live a heart-healthy life. Remember that you are your own best advocate.

Communication is the key to a successful partnership with your doctor. The three key issues to address through that partnership are these:

What is my main problem?

What do I need to do?

Why is it important for me to do this?

If you and your doctor focus on these three issues, then you'll be working together to improve your health.

— Jennifer H. Mieres, MD, Director of Nuclear Cardiology, Division of Cardiology, New York University School of Medicine

who's the best of the best, but she has a dry personality and lacks warmth, you may still choose to have her do your surgery. It's all about you getting the best medical care you can.

> *My first cardiologist was a good doctor, but he had a lousy bedside manner. After several months of being in his care I fired him.*
> —Susan, Mission Viejo, CA, age 58

Susan knew her doctor was competent to take care of her, but he lacked the warmth, care, and concern she wanted. She thought through the decision carefully and decided to find a new doctor that would better suit her needs. The message: Don't hesitate to leave a doctor if you're unhappy with the services he's providing. It's important to your health to have a good relationship with your doctor—it's too important to ignore.

FINDING A DOCTOR: WHAT ARE
YOU LOOKING FOR?

Board certification.   At the very least, you want a doctor who is board certified, which means that he or she is trained in a medical specialty area and has passed qualifying tests. Board certified physicians are required to keep up to date in their specialty by attending medical conferences, and to pass occasional recertification exams. You can call the American Board of Medical Specialists to find out whether a doctor is board certified at (866) 275–2267 or go to http://www.abms.org.

Education and training.   Try to find out where the doctor has done his/her training. Ask about medical school, residency, and fellowships, which is added training for a specialty. Many doctors post their degrees, certification, and honors on their office walls. If you don't see them, don't be embarrassed to ask. You wouldn't hesitate asking in-depth questions if you were buying a car or a house, would you? Well, these professionals are taking care of your body and your health. So ask them: Where did you get your medical degree? Where did you do your residency and fellowship? All of these are perfectly reasonable questions.

Details about the office and how things work.   Don't be shy about interviewing the doctor or office staff, and ask:

- *About office policies.* Who covers for the doctor if he or she is off or away? Who else might you see or talk to if you have a medical concern? What hospital is the doctor affiliated with? If the doctor has privileges at more than one hospital, can you go to the hospital of your choice? What are the procedures for a patient in the case of an emergency?
- *About matters of convenience and personal attention.* What are the office hours? How big is the doctor's caseload? What's the average waiting time for seeing the doctor? What is the average amount of time the doctor spends with a patient face to face? How long does it take to get an appointment? Then ask yourself: Where is the office located—is it close to where you work or live?

- *About health insurance.* Will the office accept your insurance? Does the office send in the insurance forms to your health-care plan for the visit or do you have to file them yourself?

After your first visit, assess your experience. Ask yourself whether that doctor and his office staff are right for you. Did you have to wait a long time to see the doctor? Was it simple to park, get through the paperwork, and sign in? How did the doctor treat you? Did he or she ask you important questions and then listen carefully to your response? Was it easy to understand what the doctor was saying? Is this someone you feel you can talk to in an honest and open fashion? Was he or she friendly and warm, and did he/she take the time to talk about other things besides your health condition? Was the environment welcoming and comforting? Or were you rushed? How did the doctor behave if you asked a question more than once? Think about your answers and write them down. It may take more than one visit to make a decision. That's okay; take your time. Of course, if you already know this isn't the doctor for you, then it's time to move on to someone else. Find another doctor who might be a better fit.

USING YOUR TIME WISELY

Once you've picked a physician, you still have to be realistic and recognize that you'll have a limited time to actually see the doctor. How can you optimize the time that you do spend with him or her?

- *For starters, write things down.* It's too easy to forget your questions and concerns. So keep good records. If you notice that your symptoms or conditions wax and wane, keep a health diary to track your condition and how it changes. Use your diary to write down questions for your doctor; put them in order of priority and bring the list with you to your appointment.
- *Make a list before each appointment.* Even if you don't keep a diary, before your appointment, be sure to write down any symptoms, medical concerns, or stresses in your life that may be affecting your health. Prioritize the issues you want to discuss and the questions you want to ask. Bring that list with you and follow it!

- *Keep a list of medications.* Include all of the vitamins, herbs, and supplements you take. (See page 14–17 for more details.) Always take it with you when you visit your doctor.
- *Be prepared.* Have your family's medical history and your medical history written down before your first visit to a new doctor. It will save time and energy, and you won't feel pressured to try to remember all those details on the spot. Your doctor can then keep your family and personal history in your medical records.
- *Take notes.* During your visit, write down your doctor's instructions and the answers to your questions. You might want to repeat the answers back to him or her to make sure you fully understand what was said.
- *Get someone to help you.* Better still, bring someone else along to take notes. That will give you more freedom to listen. After all, talking to your doctor involves processing a lot of information.
- *Stay informed.* Before your visit, research your medical concerns via reliable sources. Look for credible books and articles from medical journals. Get your information from universities or health centers, and connect with national organizations like WomenHeart at www.womenheart.org or www.hearthealthy-women.org. This information is likely to be the most accurate, up-to-date, and helpful to you.
- *Ask your doctor for resources and information.* At your appointment, ask your doctor for more information. You might be given pamphlets, videos, or audiotapes to review. (See the Resources section for other options.)
- *Be open.* Talk frankly with your doctor about what's going on with your health. Don't be embarrassed to tell the truth about how you feel. Your doctor can't help you if he or she doesn't know what's really going on. For instance, if you feel depressed and are having trouble following the recommended diet and exercise program, your doctor can help. He or she can refer you to a mental health professional to address your concerns. What your doctor doesn't know can ultimately hurt you. So give your doctor the information he or she needs, so he or she can be the best doctor for you. If you're having trouble being honest with your doctor, that may reflect a problem with the doctor/patient

relationship and it may be an indication that you need to find another doctor with whom you feel more comfortable.

- *Ask questions.* If you have a concern or question, don't hold back or be shy. Actively participate in the appointment. Repeat the answers back to your doctor to make sure you're accurately retaining the information. Get the input you need about the risks and benefits of recommended diagnostic tests, treatment options, and medications. If you're having a test or procedure done, ask how this will affect you in going to work, being at home, or driving. Ask about potential side effects or medical issues that could arise. Ask about the recovery period and what you can expect in terms of discomfort. If you're concerned about your insurance coverage, discuss the possible costs.

- *Talk about communication.* During your visit, talk to your doctor about the best ways to communicate outside the office. Should nonemergencies be handled by e-mail or by phone? What's the best way to reach him or her with questions? When is an office visit essential?

GETTING ANOTHER OPINION

Remember my story? I saw more than one cardiologist before I was put on the right medications—and that was the cardiologist who finally gave me my life back. But going from one doctor to another wasn't easy. I felt the way many women heart patients do—that by seeing another doctor, I'd be hurting my doctor's feelings. It's remarkable how much loyalty you can feel toward your doctor, even though your health may be deteriorating and it's clear that you're not getting the care you need. Let me tell you a bit more about my story.

I spent a lot of time on the phone with a staff person at WomenHeart talking about the fact that my health was declining. I told her I just wasn't getting any better. She kept insisting that I get another medical opinion, and encouraged me to travel to the Mayo Clinic to see a specific physician there. She kept asking: "What have you got to lose? What on earth is stopping you?" My answer was typical. "How can I leave my family to do this? I have three boys who need me and a husband who works all of the time, and no family here to take care of them. I can't leave town to see another doctor." Her response: "Well, what's your family going to do if you're no longer there at all?" That's all I needed to hear—I talked to the other doctor and scheduled an appointment. But it wasn't quite that simple. I experienced a lot of anxiety over getting another opinion about my health situation. Believe it or not, I felt guilty that somehow I was betraying my cardiologist.

I told my husband—a physician—that I didn't want my cardiologist to be upset with me for seeking another medical opinion. I said I felt like an adulterer. I think he had to hold back his frustration—and his urge to laugh. He simply said, "If your cardiologist has any problem with you getting another opinion, then he's the problem and you need to leave him anyway. Any good physician would welcome another opinion." Sure enough, my cardiologist gave me his blessing, no problem. In fact, I think he was relieved that I was getting another opinion—he no longer had to hear from me every day.

Many women heart patients report having these anxieties about getting another opinion. But the reality is this: Your health should be your primary concern, not your doctor's feelings. And if you need the eyes, ears, and hands of multiple doctors to help you recover, so be it. If your original doctor has limited experience with cases such as yours or you have concerns about any aspect of the care you're receiving, it's totally appropriate to seek another opinion. That opinion can be invaluable. Recognize that you and your family deserve the best that medicine has to offer. So be persistent, and don't hesitate to pursue a second—or third or fourth—opinion.

> *Almost a year after my heart attack and angioplasty, and after a routine nuclear stress test, my doctor told me that I needed another angioplasty and stents. I was feeling fine and was following a very strict regimen of exercise, diet, and medication. So I didn't immediately accept his diagnosis and insisted that we do additional testing. The next test was negative and when I took all of the test results to other doctors for a third and fourth opinion, they all felt that the first test did not really show a problem, but rather my breast tissue had obscured the results. It was difficult challenging my cardiologist's diagnosis, but I was glad I did.*

Nine years later I still haven't needed anything done to my heart—I feel fine.

—Irene, Springfield, NJ, age 51

By being assertive and insisting on additional medical opinions, Irene saved herself from having to go through an unnecessary procedure and all the upheaval that goes with it. My colleague on the WomenHeart staff was right: "What have you got to lose?" Or, put another way, you may have everything to gain.

LISTENING TO YOUR BODY

It took eight months for my heart problems to be accurately diagnosed. I wasn't feeling well and kept going back to my doctor telling her that something was wrong. I was tested for everything under the sun. I even had an EKG but that showed no problem. My symptoms got progressively worse—from tingling down my left arm to breathing problems to chest pain. Finally, out of desperation, she referred me for a nuclear stress test; it was positive for a heart problem. But even then the doctor still didn't believe it. So she sent me for an echocardiogram. After that test, I didn't even leave hospital. They sent me right in for bypass surgery.

—Anna, Indianapolis, IN, age 48

Anna listened and paid attention to what her body was telling her. Are you listening to what your body may be telling you? Make conscientious attempts to pay attention to how you feel. Trust your instincts and follow them. You know yourself better than anyone else does. And if you're not getting a satisfactory response to your health concerns from the health-care system, then educate yourself and pursue other options. That self-awareness, persistence, and self-advocacy can save your life.

You are your own best advocate. Search, read, and ask questions until you find the answers that you're so desperately seeking. Don't settle for anything less than straight answers to even what might seem the minutest questions. I have to continue to educate myself. I went in every direction possible in seeking the available resources to get the proper treatment, which also turned out to be the way to get an accurate diagnosis. Don't ever give up, don't ever stop asking questions!!

—Tasha, Hot Springs, AR, age 40

You may have to find a WomenHeart Center near you to get the help you need. WomenHeart Centers were created specifically to address the special needs of women heart patients. (Available centers are found on the WomenHeart Web site at http://www.womenheart.org/home_resources/resources_1.asp.) Many WomenHeart Centers are housed in teaching and research hospitals, which are an excellent option for any patient struggling to find doctors who know and use the latest medical information, technology, procedures, and treatments in the country.

Another great resource is the U.S. Department of Health and Human Services Web site, www.hospitalcompare.hhs.gov. You can find information there about hospitals in your area. It also provides tools that let you compare area hospitals, an invaluable service for health-care consumers.

WHY WOMENHEART CENTERS?

Closing the gender treatment gap by getting physicians to integrate care and follow established guidelines will require a concerted effort and a multipronged approach. We see a great need for doctors to have access to one-stop shopping for resources related to the diagnosis, treatment, and integrated management of women heart patients. That's what WomenHeart Centers provide.

When it comes to heart disease, men and women are different. Over the past five years, clinical research has repeatedly pointed out important differences in the way women perceive their own risk; the way health-care providers evaluate and treat the disease in women; and the poorer health outcomes for women in terms of both death and disability.

—Susan K. Bennett, MD, Director, Women's Heart Program,
George Washington University Hospital

Working with Your Hospital and Health Plans

Once you have heart disease, bills begin piling up almost immediately and seem to multiply on your desk. You're not even sure where some of them came from. You wonder: Are they going to bill my insurance directly or am I responsible right now? Bills can be a huge source of frustration.

> *I ranted that my medical bills were by now the better part of a foot thick! I raved that I had no time for anything but bills! My patience with health-care providers was at an end! I was ready to throttle any insurance company worker who demanded "proof of need"—as if I, a lay person, should know! And what was going on with health-care providers' offices that didn't seem to want to take the trouble to state the obvious concerning "need" to non-medical insurance blokes? I yelled in frustration and anger at the injustice that heart disease was not only threatening the life of my beloved but also requiring us, no, me to suffer through unending paperwork torture.*
>
> —Linda's husband John, DeKalb, IL, age 72

John's reaction to all of the stress over bills and dealing with uncooperative insurance companies, hospitals, and providers' offices is not unusual. It can be overwhelming to anyone caught up in it. So what can you do?

First, become informed as soon as possible. It's critical for you to know about all of your health-care plans and what you have in terms of coverage. Get on the phone with your insurance company or review the packet describing your plans, and get to know the plans' policies and procedures. If you're on Medicare call them at 1-800-medicare or go to their Web site for information, www.medicare.gov. Know what your deductibles and copays are. You don't want to have problems down the road and get caught with tremendous bills that you can't afford to pay.

As with any other element of your health-care management, it's important to be assertive and persistent when dealing with insurers. If you find that whoever you're talking to is not helpful, ask to speak to his/her supervisor. Begin going up the ladder of health-care representatives if you have to—but get the help and support you need. Try to find a "champion" health-care representative to help you—yes, they do exist! It just takes some effort to find one. It might be an administrator from the human resources department at your office; it might be the person you talk to at your health-care plan; or a staff person at your doctor's office. But whoever it is, when you find her, never let her go. If at all possible, get his or her name and a direct phone number. Let your champion know what's been going on with reimbursement between your health-care plan, the doctors' offices, or health-care facilities. Tell your champion about your health problems and the road you've been on—including the human side of your situation. Your champion will go to bat for you by empathizing with your situation and advocating on your behalf to your health-care plan. You can also speak to your human resources office at work; they can often help when you're having nightmare issues with your health-care plan. They can also help point you in the right direction to connect with the best health-care representative to talk to.

Stay in touch with your doctors' offices and the health-care facilities you've used. Talk to the people there and stay on top of what's happening with their billing process. If there's a holdup in a reimbursement, it could be their mistake. For example, if their office miscodes something, they won't get reimbursed and then you'll keep getting the bills, unnecessarily. Find an advocate in your doctors' offices and health-care facilities who will work hard to correct errors. Again, get their name and phone numbers—have them resubmit bills as needed to your carrier.

> The insurance company informed me that they were not paying a further $5,000 or so on Linda's hospital bill because the company had decided to perform an audit of the hospital's billing and other procedures. That was it—I went to a senior billing person at the hospital to straighten this out. She called me back with joyous news that the audit had indeed been completed months before and they were just waiting for the check to be cut. Grrrrr!
>
> —Linda's husband, John, DeKalb, IL, age 72

John was assertive with the hospital and the health-insurance plan, and that's how he ultimately solved the problems concerning his wife's hospital and doctor bills, which were extensive. But he wasn't spared the frustration and anxiety that comes with such a process.

SURVIVAL TIPS FOR DEALING WITH INSURERS

- Be patient.
- Keep copies of every scrap of paper from every doctor, hospital, or ambulance ride. Set up a file system that works for you to keep track of all the paper.
- Know what your benefit handbook says.
- Have all pertinent details of your insurance coverage in mind and your handbook available.
- Have your Explanation of Benefits and bills available when talking to the insurers, doctors' offices, hospitals, or other providers of care.
- Keep a paper trail, write down the dates and times of every phone call, person you talk to, and information that was given to you.
- Find out how to appeal your case, just in case you need to.
- Keep track of appeal limitations.
- Keep in fairly constant touch with providers until the final bills have been paid.
- Be aware that Medicare and other payers may have different fiscal years, which affect deductibles.
- Be aware that Medicare may not inform your commercial insurance carrier if it denies a claim. In addition, your insurance company may take no action until you request it.

—Linda's husband, John, DeKalb, IL, age 72

If you're having trouble with a hospital, try contacting the ombudsman. A hospital ombudsman can act as your advocate, but in a limited capacity—because they do represent the hospital's interests. Nonetheless, it's worth it to involve an ombudsman if you're having trouble getting the hospital to cooperate with you, with your doctors, or your health plans.

Over time, if you can't resolve insurance issues and the bills simply aren't being paid by your health-insurance company, you have several options:

- Send in an appeal to your state insurance commissioner. To locate your state insurance commissioner, go to: http://www.naic.org/state_web_map.htm

- Contact state regulatory agencies for help. To find the local agency that regulates insurance in your state, go to: www.ambest.com/directory/govdir.html?l=1&Menu=Industry+Resources,State+Insurance+Regulators
- Patient advocacy groups can help you with insurance-related problems. They can also give you detailed information on how to support your appeal. You can find relevant information at www.womenheart.org, or go to www.patientadvocate.org.
- If you're having trouble with a managed care company covering a treatment or procedure, visit www.aarp.org/health/insurance/managed_care/a2003-04-22-hmoappeal.html for more detailed information on how to appeal your case.
- See the Resources section for additional information.

THE FINAL CHAPTER

WomenHeart saved my life. And I'm not alone. Many women heart patients find the solace and support they need to get through heart disease by connecting with other women heart patients. They feel compelled to join advocacy groups, so other women won't have to endure what they've been through. The last chapter of this book shares information on how you can become an advocate—an experience that can both transform you and help others. Advocacy makes a difference and you can feel it, see it, and experience it.

chapter ten

BECOMING AN ADVOCATE FOR CHANGE
The Bigger Picture

*Many persons have a wrong idea of what
constitutes true happiness.
It is not attained through self-gratification but
through fidelity to a worthy purpose.*
—Helen Keller

Helen Keller has always been one of my heroes! She took a horrific experience growing up and devoted her life to a worthy cause—changing the way the world viewed the blind and deaf—through her determination, passion, and heart. That's what activism is—recognizing that some ill in the world exists and bringing about systemwide social or political change. Advocacy is just organized activism.

I never thought in a million years that I'd be where I am today. The idea of becoming an advocate for women with heart disease never even crossed my mind. Sometimes I think that life takes you down certain unexpected paths for a reason—and here I am. Over the past four years or so, there's been a dramatic change in the level of activism among women with heart disease. In the past, it wasn't easy to get women involved—they seemed elusive and unsure. Now they're front and center, thousands of them. They're acting as advocates, and involved in outreach, community education, and support activities around the issue of women and heart disease. Numerous nonprofit coalition groups, businesses, the media, many states, and the federal government have all come on board. Thousands of people are out there working tirelessly; and I've been lucky enough to watch this major shift unfold before my eyes.

The stigma seems to be lifting. Women with heart disease are coming forward and wanting to make a difference. They're ready and able to see the larger picture, and demand change on behalf of all of the women who can't advocate for themselves. Maybe you'll join us. Let's explore the issue.

> *The first time I was taken to the hospital, the emergency room cardiologist did an EKG and a blood test, then told me I was just having an anxiety attack and sent me home. Fortunately, my primary physician gave me more tests and then sent me to another cardiologist for a stress test, which led to an angiogram and angioplasty. A few months later I dialed 911 and a fireman came and put an oxygen mask on my face, but he told my husband that he didn't turn on the oxygen because he thought I was just having an anxiety attack. Well, I ended up with another angiogram and stent. Another time I was having symptoms and I called 911. This time I was home alone and the fire department didn't take me seriously again. The fireman said, "You seem very anxious. Did you have an argument with your husband this morning?" I said, "Yes, I am anxious—I know my body and I am having a cardiac event and I'm in serious trouble!" That day I went to the hospital for my triple bypass!*
>
> —Marilyn, Palm Desert, CA, age 62

Unfortunately, Marilyn is not alone. There are thousands of women like her in this country who are misdiagnosed, or experience delayed diagnosis, mistreatment, or inadequate treatment for their hearts. We lose our mothers, grandmothers, sisters, and aunts every year because of the ignorance and lack of education of others, including doctors and healthcare workers. Every year, for the past twenty years, more women in the United States have died of heart disease then men. This is a situation that should make all of us angry.

The good news is that women in this country are beginning to understand the issues surrounding heart disease—including the fact that it's

DOES ADVOCACY REALLY CHANGE THINGS?

I've worked in the field of women's health advocacy for twenty years. My firm, Bass & Howes, working with the Congressional Caucus for Women's Issues, was the catalyst for turning women's health issues into a political issue. In 1990, we drafted legislation that Congress passed requiring women to be included in clinical trials. Of course, the most egregious examples of the exclusion were in the area of women and heart disease. Much has changed in twenty years and it's because women's voices are now heard in the halls of Congress and the rooms of the White House.

I am personally so proud of what women with heart disease have accomplished. Although there is still a long way to go, science now supports the fact that heart disease in women is different from heart disease in men, and that represents a seismic change in medicine in very a short period of time. This would not have happened without women's personal stories and advocacy prodding public policy makers, scientists, and clinicians.

—Joanne Howes, Partner, DDB Issues & Advocacy

the number one health threat they face. Awareness of that fact has risen dramatically in recent years—from 30 percent awareness among women in 1997, to 57 percent awareness in 2004.[1] But those statistics also tell us that we have a lot of work to do. They show that there are a significant number of women in the United States who don't know heart disease is their greatest health risk. And, among women who do know it, most don't think that it will strike them—only 13 percent recognize that they, personally, are at risk. Many women are simply unaware that they have risk factors for heart disease. But the reality is that 80 percent of women between the ages of forty and sixty have one or more risk factors, so they're at increased risk of developing heart disease.[2]

---

1. L. Mosca, H. Mochari, A. Christian, et al., "National Study of Women's Awareness, Preventive Action and Barriers to Cardiovascular Health," *Circulation* 113 (2006): 525–34.

2. Ibid.; L. Mosca, W. K. Jones, K. B. King, et al., "Awareness, Perception and Knowledge of Heart Disease Risk and Prevention Among Women in the United States," *Archives of Family Medicine* 9 (2000): 506–15.

Three doctors assured me that my irregular heart beat was nor-
mal, but I wasn't so sure. So I went to the Mayo Clinic at Scotts-
dale. They told me that I needed further testing. The fifth doctor I
saw finally diagnosed my need for surgery. I ended up needing
five-way bypass surgery. Until then, I'd never been told or knew
that I had heart disease.

—Jane, Bayside, CA, age 62

These kinds of situations tell us why so many women heart patients are becoming advocates. We believe that women have the right to receive early detection, accurate diagnosis, and proper treatment for their hearts. Advocates who work and volunteer for groups like the American Heart Association, the Heart Truth Campaign, and WomenHeart are speaking in national and local forums. They're actively and persistently getting the word out to anyone who will listen. They're helping the public, the media, government, businesses, and health-care professionals understand the issues that face women with heart disease, and how to improve aware-ness and educate those women who haven't heard the message or don't yet own the message. Even though we've come a long way in a few years, why is it that so many women still have heart problems that go unde-tected, or aren't properly diagnosed and treated? Why is it that so many women still aren't getting the care they deserve?

Most people—and many physicians—still don't realize that heart dis-ease is an equal-opportunity killer. As a result, women are less likely to recognize the symptoms early and seek treatment, they're less likely to be accurately diagnosed, and they're less likely to get appropriate care. For one thing, women often don't present with the classic symptoms of heart disease. For another, heart disease is a different animal in women—in part, because of hormonal issues and the difference in size of women's vessels. Historically, treatments have been standardized on men, be-cause, until the mid–1990s, women were not included in clinical trials. And even today women are underrepresented in heart-related research studies—they comprise only 25 percent of the participants.[3] As a result, most doctors are forced to treat women using adapted diagnostic proce-dures and treatments that were originally developed for men—and that can lead to treatment by trial and error.

---

3. http://www.womenheart.org/information/women_and_heart_disease_fact_sheet.asp

When I initially entered the ER, I was ignored for almost an hour. Well, that's not quite true—they ran a toxicology test for cocaine because they thought I might have abused illegal drugs. I guess that's what would be the first impression when you see a very young black female with no socks and shoes, unkempt hair, and no pocketbook or identification. After begging and complaining of chest pain—and my dad getting really angry—an EKG was finally done! A few minutes later I was moved to a private room so that I could be placed on monitors and observation equipment. I had a massive heart attack, was transferred to another facility twenty-four hours later, followed by quintuple bypass surgery two days after that. I was denied cardiac rehabilitation and recovered at home for three months. I'm lucky to be alive.

—Sarah, West Hempstead, NY, age 29

WHY SHOULD YOU GET INVOLVED?

Sarah's story is compelling and disturbing. It illustrates what many women go through. Consider the need for education. As the baby boom generation ages—with its 77 million people—more and more women will have to confront the issues that accompany heart disease. Consider the statistics.[4]

---

4. U. S. Department of Labor, Training, and Employment Information Notice No. 12–00, "Older Workers: Aging Baby Boomers and Their Implications for Employment and Training Programs," February 27, 2001.

Age: 2000, Census 2000 Brief, U.S. Department of Commerce, Economics and Statistics Administration, U.S. Census Bureau. Issued October 2001.

Marketresearch.com, Executive Summary, "The Market for Boomers Turning 50," August 1, 1998.

Y. J. Gist, and L. I. Hetzel, "We the People: Aging in the United States," Census 2000 Special Report, U.S. Department of Commerce, Economics, and Statistics Administration, U.S. Census Bureau. Issued December 2004.

Daphne Spain, PhD, "Societal Trends: The Aging Baby Boom and Women's Increased Independence," Final report prepared for the Federal Highway Administration, U.S. Department of Transportation, Order No. DTFH61–97-P–00314, December 1997.

"United States Aging Demographics," prepared by the UNC Institute on Aging, 2000.

Every day, more women enter the at-risk group.

- In the 2000 census, the baby boom fueled a 55 percent increase in the number of people fifty to fifty-four years old, the largest increase of any age cohort. The second largest was forty to forty-nine years old.
- Every seven seconds another baby boomer turns fifty. That's more than 12,000 people a day.
- According to a 2004 study by Kalorama Information, the next ten years will see an accelerating market for cardiovascular therapeutics.[5] Based on the study, in 2004, the population over forty-five years of age represented approximately 36 percent of the total U.S. population, but almost 90 percent of cases of cardiovascular disease. In 2013, more than 40 percent of the U.S. population will be over forty-five—and represent 95 percent of cardiovascular disease cases.
- In addition, rising rates of obesity and Type II diabetes—both of which are major risk factors for heart disease—suggest that this is the women's health issue that will become even more compelling in the years ahead.
- Within the next ten years, it's estimated that there will be more than 16 million women in the United States living with heart disease.

Women are living longer.

- The average life expectancy today is age seventy-six—and women live longer than men do.
- In 2000, according to the U.S. Census, there were more than 20 million women over age sixty-five in the U.S. compared to 14 million men.

Baby boomers strive for a more youthful lifestyle than past generations—and advocacy can play an important educational role.

---

5. News Release, Kalorama Information, "Cardiovascular Therapeutics Find Huge Market in Aging Baby Boomers," March 9, 2004.

- More women are likely to confront heart disease and strive for a healthful recovery.
- More women will be seeking guidance on how to live a long, full life with the disease.
- There is a dramatic difference in the female experience with heart disease, and there are few resources for women to help them thrive in the face of that experience.

Heart disease represents a major health threat for women—and by taking action, we can help prevent unnecessary deaths.

- Cardiovascular disease is the number one killer of men and women. For women that means 367,000 deaths each year.
- In terms of total deaths, according to the Alliance for Aging Research, heart disease has claimed the lives of more women than men every year since 1984. That may be due in part to the fact that women are less likely to recognize a heart event and seek treatment.
- Women receive only 33 percent of angioplasties, stents, and bypass surgeries, and only 28 percent of implantable defibrillators.[6]

By 2015, according to the Alliance for Aging Research, all the baby boomers will be over fifty years old, and the oldest will begin to reach sixty-five. Just think of the impact you can make on women and their families—by being there for them, by educating them, by advocating on their behalf!

WHAT CAN ADVOCACY DO FOR YOU?

With no one to talk to, I felt so alone. It wasn't until my cardiologist recommended I try the WomenHeart Web site that I realized there were other women who were experiencing the same feelings as me—that's when I knew I wasn't alone. As I got stronger, I

---

6. Women and Heart Disease Fact Sheet available online at
www.womenheart.org/information/women_and_heart_disease_fact_sheet.asp.

wanted to reach out to other women who were living with heart disease. Truthfully, I didn't expect to become as involved as I am, but my advocacy work has become my life's passion. It's truly changed my life.

—Joann, Huntington Station, NY, age 59

Becoming an advocate is transformational. It's therapeutic. It helps you to think beyond yourself and your own issues. You'll touch the lives of women and their families. You'll be a woman who informs, inspires, and empowers others to make changes in their lifestyle choices that can literally save their lives. Being involved gives you hope—for the women who come after you—for your children and grandchildren in the next generations. Your involvement will make the world a better place. And you'll be surprised where it will take you. Volunteering and getting involved challenges your own self-created boundaries. It's a tremendous challenge to stretch those boundaries and reach your own potential—advocacy gives you the opportunity.

I knew I wanted to help other women heart patients, and advocate for them and myself. I found that a kind word is worth a million bucks—that it helps other women heart patients a lot to talk when they're going through a hard time. It's so much fun seeing the change in the faces of women heart patients as soon as they realize that they're no longer alone—that we're in this together. Over time they laugh, open up, talk about their experiences with heart disease, and ask questions, all of which helps them in their recovery. I meet women heart patients every day because I get calls from the hospital to help the ones who are struggling with their heart events. It gives me great pleasure to be an advocate and helping others.

—Alice, Kenduskeag, ME, age 66

Many women heart patients feel isolated and alone. But by reaching out, you can make the powerful connection to others that is so important to your recovery. Through the process of being an advocate, you also become an advocate for yourself. You can learn important life lessons. And that, in turn, can ignite a passion for living that heals on many levels.

THE HEALING POWER OF ADVOCACY

It's been my observation that participation in advocacy organizations can accelerate a woman's post-event recovery process exponentially through the healing powers of connection and the subsequent activation of positive feelings that relate directly to physical health. Through advocacy, women are emotionally supported and encouraged to talk about their traumatic events and to tell their stories.

Sharing in a safe and compassionate social environment has a profound therapeutic effect that enables people to reduce or extinguish fearful emotions, increase healthful positive emotions, integrate their experience into their psyche and move forward in life. Advocacy provides myriad opportunities to become actively involved in self-healing and to take control of one's health issues, while simultaneously helping others. Feelings of powerlessness, shown to significantly increase stress and therefore heart risk, begin to dissolve and are replaced with empowered states of mind and behaviors. This eliminates the traditional feminine conflict of self-care versus care of others—as self-empowerment is shared and inspires self-care in others. Many people go well beyond reclaiming pre-event functioning and blossom in previously underdeveloped ways.

Dean Ornish, pioneering cardiologist, has said that our hearts are more than a pump—that we also have an emotional, psychological, and spiritual heart. I believe the success of advocacy lies in the healing of the whole heart as described by Ornish through profound connectedness and the activation of healing states within compassionate, attuned, and resonant relationships.

—Kimberly Kiddoo, PhD, Psychologist, Coral Gables, FL

During that time I asked a lot of questions, I wanted to understand what was going on in my body, and why the tests and procedures were necessary. I advocated for myself—I felt so empowered. I was so proud of the strong woman that I'd become—such a contrast to the way I felt following my heart attack. Thanks to my advocacy work, I've experienced a positive change in my knowledge, attitude, and behavior as a woman living with heart disease.

—Joann, Huntington Station, NY, age 59

Of course, change is not easy and when you decide to do advocacy work, you might find some resistance from your friends, family, and society. There's always push back when you take a stand, and you might experience negativity from people you least expect. After all, you'll be questioning the status quo. You'll be getting noticed. What you say and do will produce a reaction—and it won't always be positive.

I'll never forget when WomenHeart decided to use my photograph for a campaign to raise awareness of the issues surrounding women and heart disease. The image showed me in a white blouse that reveals my scar. I asked my sons and husband whether they were okay with it. My oldest son, Ben, gave his approval without a second thought. My middle son, Nathaniel, said, after some thought, "You know what? This is a beautiful photograph and you've got to do it." My youngest son, Jon, said, "Yeah, it's okay if you do it as long as no one really knows who you are or your name. I don't want to be embarrassed." My husband said, "Of course, you have to do it. It's okay for all of the husbands in the world to be jealous of me!" Well, unfortunately for Jon, my white blouse ad, PSA, and name have been plastered all over the media locally and nationally. I was so worried about him when that happened. But the first time he saw it, he came home and said, "Mom, it's all right. Actually, my friends really like the picture and especially like what you're trying to do." Well, I almost burst out crying with relief from those words of acceptance.

Of course, when you put yourself and your opinions out there in public, the responses can range from being very supportive to being downright rude. When you're an advocate, you have to expect some flack. So brace yourself. In my experience, it's been worth it—because positive social, medical and political changes are happening. It's helped women who have heart disease and it's helping women who don't. Most importantly, the cause has and will continue to save precious lives.

IT DOES A WORLD OF GOOD

The fellowship that comes with advocacy can be very valuable to women who want to live well with heart disease. Advocates are making a difference and that's good for their hearts! Many women heart patients gain something from the experience, as evidenced by the fact that advocacy is on the rise. For example, WomenHeart membership has increased from

4,000 in 2001 to 16,000 today—and it's growing rapidly. Over the past year, nearly four million women have visited the WomenHeart Web site for resources and support.

> *My lifestyle has been dramatically altered [since my heart event] and I was severely depressed until I found an advocacy organiza- tion to join. Then I realized that I was not alone! Now I've formed a support group, which has greatly enhanced my life by giving me the opportunity to help others. My mission is to encourage women to be vigilant in pursuing a proper diagnosis. After all, we know our bodies better than anyone!*
>
> —Linda, Kenosha, WI, age 46

There's no question that there's power in numbers. Together we really can make a difference. Your voice is strong and far-reaching—and you have a host of advocacy options from which to choose. What can you do?

- Join an advocacy organization or support network in your area.
- Join a national organization.
- Help other heart patients by forming a support group.
- Raise awareness through community outreach and education; by giving media interviews or public speeches; or by spearheading events.
- Work with and advise the health-care community.
- Affect public policy by talking to your representatives in Con- gress and your state legislature about policy issues, by talking to the press, and through community activism.
- Remember, any volunteer effort matters. You can answer phones, stuff envelopes, put up posters for upcoming events, or work on a committee. All volunteers are welcome.

> *I have always tried to find the good in things, and finally I'm able to find the good in having heart disease. I was meant to meet my cardiologist, to work at the center, to start a support group, and then to become an active supporter of an advocacy organization. I'm making lemonade out of lemons. My relationships are stronger and healthier. I try not to get caught up in pettiness, it*

just wastes everyone's energy. I have grown and I have been blessed by it all. It is only in retrospect that I realized all of these things. While going through it, I definitely felt alone and afraid. Now I feel alive, happy, and empowered.

—Claire, La Costa, CA, age 53

CHOICES CHOICES CHOICES

Here are three major organizations that offer programs you can become involved with:

- *The American Heart Association* (AHA). Founded in 1924, the American Heart Association is one of the world's premier health organizations. The American Heart Association supports research, health promotion and disease prevention, access to quality health care, and an advocacy agenda. Since 2003, the organization has focused on women's heart health as an important issue with the creation of Go Red Campaign. With local branches, an advocacy director, and an advocacy committee in every state, the AHA has the organization in place to influence legislation at the state level. These committees are made up of physicians, stroke and heart disease survivors, physical education specialists, community leaders, research scientists, and key volunteers from the organization's *You're the Cure* network (see page 218), which serves as a first response unit when key issues are considered by lawmakers at the state level. The AHA has a similar structure at the federal level—although it's a far bigger organization. The AHA can help you host an event, become an advocate, and stay in tune with major legislative activities. Local branches have their own specific activities, including—in some cases—educational events for women or specific ethnic groups; they also do a lot of fund-raising activities. For more information or to locate your local branch, visit www.americanheart.org.
- *The Heart Truth Campaign.* The Heart Truth is a national awareness campaign designed to educate women about heart disease. It's sponsored by the National Heart, Lung, and Blood Institute (NHLBI), which is part of the National Institutes of Health. De-

signed to warn women that heart disease is the number one health threat they face, the campaign introduced the Red Dress as the national symbol for women and heart disease awareness in 2003 to deliver an urgent wake-up call to American women. The Red Dress is designed to remind women of the need to protect their heart health and inspire them to take action. NHLBI continues to lead the nation in a landmark heart-health awareness movement that is being embraced by millions who share the common goal of spreading the word about heart disease and promoting better heart health for all women. The Heart Truth Campaign also sponsors outreach and advocacy training. For more information, visit www.nhlbi.nih.gov/health/hearttruth.

- *WomenHeart: The National Coalition for Women with Heart Disease.* WomenHeart serves a unique purpose nationally by aiming to improve the quality of life and health care of women with heart disease through its support, education, and advocacy activities. WomenHeart offers everything from online support to local support networks, to science and leadership development programs to advocacy training and a biannual National Membership Conference. You can work at a community level or at a national level. The WomenHeart website offers a tremendous menu of options for women with heart disease and their families, which includes information of up-to-date medical news, fitness and wellness, and links to other resources in the community and beyond. Find out more at www.womenheart.org.

Becoming an Advocate

I've always been a driven, high-energy person and very optimistic. Through my training at the Science and Leadership Symposium I learned a lot. I joined WomenHeart in their efforts to reach out to other women heart patients. Over time, I became the Support Network Regional Coordinator for the Great Lakes. It's very helpful to share your feelings and thoughts with other women heart patients. I'm proving that I'm still that same vivacious woman I've always been. I just happen to have heart disease.

—Pat, Lansing, MI, age 74

LEARNING MORE HELPS YOU BECOME
YOUR OWN BEST ADVOCATE

Now for an interesting story. My sister Teresa came home from the Women-Heart Biannual Membership Meeting and immediately made an appointment with her primary care doctor to get a cardiac referral. Her labs are good but she is obese and is being treated for high cholesterol and high blood pressure. So she tells the doctor she wants a referral to cardiology for a nuclear stress test. The doctor says to her, "We don't do nuclear stress tests just on anyone. You can get just a regular stress test." My sister tells the doctor, "Don't waste my time." The doctor then says, "You don't have any risk factors!" My sister says, "Excuse me, I had bypass surgery in my leg ten years ago from calcification; my sister had a heart attack at age forty-three; my father passed away at age fifty-six from a heart attack; his father died at age forty-three and his mother at age forty-two. My maternal grandmother had a pacemaker, congestive heart failure, and was a diabetic, and then died from a brain tumor at age eighty-six. Exactly which risk factor were you looking for?" Then she started spouting Women-Heart statistics at this female doctor. Obviously she got the referral to the cardiologist and the doctor got the name of the WomenHeart Web site. So another success story. This time from the meeting!

—Eileen, on behalf of her sister Teresa, Manassas, VA, ages 53 and 54

There are a great many advocacy training options. The choice of advocacy activities is up to you, but I strongly recommend that you go through a training program offered through an organization such as the American Heart Association, the Heart Truth Campaign, or WomenHeart. They can give you the tools you need to become a more effective advocate, which in turn will make a greater impact and give you the opportunity to reach more people. Here are the advocacy training and development programs they offer:

- *The American Heart Association (AHA) You're the Cure*. You can become involved in the advocacy initiatives of the AHA through the *You're the Cure* Advocacy Network (www.americanheart.org/yourethecure). This system allows interested people to be con-

tacted electronically via e-mail when AHA priority issues are being considered at any level of government. *You're the Cure* advocates then respond to their individual legislators either via
e-mail, phone call, letter, fax, or personal visit, depending on the
situation. Go to http://www.americanheart.org/presenter
.jhtml?identifier=2945 to get more information on how you can
get involved with the varied activities of the AHA. For more information from the AHA about women and heart disease, go to
www.goredforwomen.org or call 1-888-MY-HEART.

- *Heart Truth Campaign's* Know the Heart Truth is a program that
reaches out to the communities that are at the greatest risk of
developing heart disease. In a train-the-trainer forum, The Heart
Truth Campaign staff equips health educators, women's health
advocates, nurses, and others invested in promoting women's
health with information and resources to spread the message
about women and heart disease in their local community. They
become champions in the community, helping to raise awareness
at the local level. Contact partners@hearttruth.org to find out if
there's a program in your city. You can always put your name on
a list for future training.

- *WomenHeart Science and Leadership Symposium.* If you're interested in becoming a spokesperson, this is a good way to learn
more about heart disease, as well as how to talk to the media
and speak publicly. Held each year at the Mayo Clinic in
Rochester, Minnesota, the Science and Leadership Symposium
is a four-day leadership training conference for a select number
of heart patients. Participants must apply for the program, where
they learn the basics of heart disease in women, including diagnosis and treatments, self-care, heart healthy nutrition, and public speaking and media training. They then return to their
communities as WomenHeart spokeswomen, where they're required to conduct a minimum of twenty-four hours of community service over a six-month period.

- *WomenHeart Advocacy Institute.* This is the next level of training for
WomenHeart members who want to become advocates. Gradu-
ates of the organization's Science and Leadership Symposium are
eligible to attend this biannual, four-day advocacy training

program in Washington, D.C. There they learn how the policy process works, and how to influence state and federal lawmakers. The institute culminates with Capitol Hill visits to Senate and House offices where participants meet with legislators and their senior health-care staff to discuss issues relating to women and heart disease, such as inclusion of more women in NIH's cardiac research studies. They return home as trained advocates, able to work with lawmakers at the state and federal level.

When I received information in the mail about the upcoming Advocacy Institute at first I thought, not me! I didn't feel that I was adequately informed about political "stuff." Then I thought: Why not? I'm a front to back reader of the newspaper, and I pride myself on at least having an idea about what's going on in my community and in the country. Plus I've never lacked for an opinion. I didn't have the knowledge about becoming an advocate, but the institute gave me the tools and showed me the way. I found myself in Washington, D.C., and loving every minute of the sessions. After we'd learned enough so we wouldn't embarrass ourselves, they turned us loose on Capitol Hill. It was fun meeting our congressmen. And stating our mission was very empowering. They actually listened to us!

—Diana, Des Moines, IA, age 55

Helping Other Heart Patients: WomenHeart Support Networks

Women heart patients want emotional and social support, but as they define it—not as someone else defines it. Women heart patients need a variety of supports at different phases during their recovery; and WomenHeart's Support Networks offer a menu of different activities that respond to the woman's individual needs. A support network can reinforce the motivation to make changes for a healthier lifestyle and serve as an educational forum for information about heart disease and treatments.

In addition to in-person support, WomenHeart provides phone and e-mail buddies for women in areas of the country where

there's no network in place. Talking on the phone and being a pen
pal has brought confidence and new friendships to many women.

—Marie Warshauer, Support Network Program Director

Research studies consistently report that patients who receive social support, and have supportive friends and family members, do better physically and emotionally, have fewer relapses and less physical suffering, and enjoy a better quality of life. They are also less isolated and less prone to depression. Mutual support—between and among patients—works because they share a common experience and with understanding of heart disease.

The WomenHeart Support Network program provides grass-roots information and support to women with heart disease through a variety of activities, such as support-group meetings, walking excursions, e-mail buddies, lunch groups, spirituality groups, and meetings with expert guest speakers. Women who participate in support network activities report they feel less isolated, more in charge of their heart disease, and more hopeful about the future. There are now forty networks around the country, led by trained WomenHeart volunteers who meet annually for additional training. For information on support networks in your area or how to start one of your own, visit http://www.womenheart .org/city_support_network.asp.

We started a WomenHeart Support Network, which has thrived
over the years. I also switched careers and am now a cardiac re-
hab nurse. This gives me so many opportunities to advocate for
women with heart disease as I interact daily with women prepar-
ing for heart surgery, recovering from a heart event, or getting
help with lifestyle management issues. Furnishing women with
information and putting a face on heart disease—someone they
can relate to—is powerful and motivating. The camaraderie of
sharing your anxieties with someone who has "walked in your
shoes" is invaluable. My advocacy continues as I spread the
word through presentations to the community, participation in
health-fair screenings, networking with other health-care
providers, and monthly outreach through our WomenHeart Net-
work meetings. The circle continues to widen, and all of us are

spreading the word about women and heart disease. From my own life-threatening event, I have seen life-changing events occur as my fellow survivors join in our shared mission to fight this number one killer of women.

—Annie, Miami, FL, age 59

SPREADING THE WORD: THE HEART TRUTH CAMPAIGN

Sometimes the simplest statements are the strongest. You can get involved in the Heart Truth Campaign by simply wearing red on National Wear Red Day or by bringing the campaign to your community. The purpose: to increase awareness that heart disease is the number one health risk for American women.

- *Raise awareness by bringing the red dresses to your community.* The Heart Truth's Red Dress "Single City" program provides the opportunity to have a traveling exhibit of designer Red Dresses come to your community as part of a women's heart-health awareness event. Host a Red Dress–themed event, such as a health fair, gala, dance, celebrity tea, power breakfast, or fashion show to benefit and promote women's heart health.
- *Celebrate National Wear Red Day.* Spearheaded by NHLBI, National Wear Red Day is held every year on the first Friday in February to build awareness for women's heart health. Make plans to participate by wearing red, organize an event and wearing a Red Dress Pin—the national symbol for women and heart disease awareness (available at http://emall.nhlbihin.net/product2 .asp?sku=56–075N).
- For information about these and other *Heart Truth* programs, visit www.hearttruth.gov, or contact partners@hearttruth.org.

WAYS TO RAISE AWARENESS AT YOUR WORKPLACE

February 3 is National Wear Red Day. In support of the National Heart, Lung, and Blood Institute's Heart Truth Campaign, National Wear Red Day is cosponsored by WomenHeart and the American Heart Association. It's designed to raise awareness of issues surrounding women and heart disease. Here are some special things you can do on February 3:

- Have everyone come to work in red: Red ties, shoes, hats, dresses, jewelry, lipstick, or wear a Red Dress Pin (available at emall.nhlbihin.net/product2.asp?sku=56-075N).
- Have speakers come and talk about the issues that face women with heart disease and how to prevent it. To find a speaker, contact your local WomenHeart Support Network, American Heart Association office, or a women's hospital in your area.
- Decorate your office in red. Go wild and have fun!
- Serve tasty, heart-healthy food for lunch. Have a cooking demonstration.
- Organize a fundraising event for WomenHeart or the American Heart Association. Be creative. Give people an incentive: Have employees wear jeans for the day (with something red, of course) and invite them to donate money for the privilege. Or hold a company-wide walkathon or stepathon competition. Challenge each other to get out there to become heart healthy through exercise and proper diet.
- Hold a CPR day at your office. Bring in someone from the American Heart Association to teach and train all employees. For more information on how, contact 1-877-AHA-4CPR or visit www.americanheart.org/presenter.jhtml?identifier=3034322.
- Hold a health fair and/or workshop for your office or company that addresses subjects such as how to reduce and manage the risk factors for heart disease. Your local branch of the American Heart Association can help you by providing support materials.

The American Heart Association, the Heart Truth Campaign, or WomenHeart can help you by providing support materials. For contact information, see the Resources section.

ADVOCACY WITH POLICY MAKERS

If you want a real challenge, working with policy makers is probably your cup of tea. It takes skill and training—and a national organization can

REACHING WOMEN OF COLOR

Because women of color are disproportionately affected by heart disease, the Heart Truth program has formed partnerships with leading national organizations representing African American and Hispanic women to sound a red alert about the nation's number one killer. Together with its partners, the campaign is engaging in national and local activities to help more women of color understand the Heart Truth—and inspire them to take action to reduce their risk for heart disease. A faith-based initiative targeted to First Ladies of the Church is one way that the Heart Truth is reaching women where they pray. If you're interested in becoming involved in this campaign, visit http://www.nhlbi.nih.gov/health/hearttruth/partners/faith_based_toolkit.htm.

train you to do the work most effectively. Once you're trained, you become the face and voice of women with heart disease. It becomes important to educate yourself about the government regulations, laws, and policies that have a direct impact on women with heart disease. If you have a story to tell, don't minimize its impact. Your words can shape the way policy makers think about women and heart disease—your story can tell them how their decisions can affect the health of their constituents. You have the right and responsibility to ask Congress and your state legislators to use your tax dollars on the issues that directly affect women and heart disease. So it's important to keep current on the issues. As of the end of 2006, these are the key issues facing us. But remember, this list is fluid and changes over time:

- Adequate growth and funding for research programs of the National Institutes of Health (NIH) and the National Heart, Lung, and Blood Institute (NHLBI) to assure that monies are designated for heart-disease research in women and for the Heart Truth campaign. Women need to be included in all phases of clinical trials and not be excluded based on sex, ethnicity, and other demographics. Funding will preferably be targeted to the ten most significant unanswered research questions related to women and heart disease—those identified in the 10 Q Report (see page 226).

- All Americans have the right to have access to quality health care. This means Medicare and Medicaid recipients should not meet obstacles in gaining access to appropriate emergency care, diagnosis, and treatment. And programs related to risk-factor modification, education, and prevention should be easily accessible. Heart patients should have unimpeded access to the full range of medications, to new medical devices and technologies, and to cardiac-rehabilitation programs. Clear, meaningful, and strong legislation should exist regarding a Patient Bill of Rights.
- The Federal Trade Commission (FTC) should ensure that there is accurate and consistent labeling of food products under the Food and Drug Administration (FDA) and the U.S. Department of Agriculture (USDA). There needs to be federal and state support for nutrition education and the promotion of exercise through appropriate government agencies. In addition, the FDA should ensure that prescription-drug labeling reflects important differences between women and men, and be based on appropriate gender differences found in clinical trials.
- The state and federal government should support "quit smoking" campaigns, and allocate funds for smoking prevention, smoking cessation programs, and antismoking educational campaigns targeted to girls and women. The government should cease financial support for the tobacco industry and help tobacco farmers find other economic alternatives.

BUILDING RELATIONSHIPS WITH POLICY MAKERS

In advocacy work, you must get to know your congressional leaders and state legislators so you can influence them to pay attention to the issues you want addressed. Relationship building is key, and that takes time and energy. As you go through this process, it's important to remember: Policy makers work for you and the heart patients you represent. Always keep that in mind.

Here's an example of relationship building: I met Senate Majority Leader Bill Frist (R-TN) at a heart-related publicity event at the U.S. Capitol. I approached him, and told him a bit about my story and my advocacy work for women with heart disease. Of course, Bill Frist is from

THE 10 Q REPORT

Each year, heart disease claims the lives of more women than men, and women heart patients continue to experience misdiagnoses, inadequate treatments, and even the wrong treatments for their conditions. On February 14, 2006, WomenHeart and the Society for Women's Health Research (SWHR), with Representatives Ginny Brown-Waite (R-Fla.) and Hilda Solis (D-Calif.), cochairs of the Congressional Caucus for Women's Issues, released a groundbreaking report on Capitol Hill. *The 10 Q Report: Advancing Women's Heart Health Through Improved Research, Diagnosis, and Treatment* identifies the top ten unanswered questions related to the development, diagnosis, and treatment of heart disease in women. Answering these questions through targeted research could cut the number of women who die prematurely of heart disease by 50 percent over the next decade. The report lays out a blueprint for a research agenda that can also help save American taxpayers millions of dollars in inappropriate and misdirected health-care costs, as well as give doctors the knowledge they need to properly treat the disease.

For more information about The 10 Q Report, go to http://www.women heart.org/10_Q_Report_06.asp.

Tennessee. And when I told him that I lived in Tennessee—voila! He took my story—and the surrounding issues—to the Senate floor and then put the related speech on his Web site for the entire world to see. Since then, Senator Frist has endorsed the 10 Q Report and supported the important messages that Congress needs to hear about women and heart disease. My very personal story—of misdiagnosis and difficulties getting the proper medical treatment—helped bring to life the compelling issues that face women with heart disease. That, combined with Senator Frist's background as a cardiovascular surgeon and the data supporting the need for more research funding and new legislation around these issues, made an impact. It never would have happened if we hadn't made that one-on-one connection.

Here are some ideas for how to build and massage relationships with policy makers so you can make a difference:

- Volunteer on a campaign for your congressional leaders and state legislators. Get others to participate as well.
- Visit your policy makers at their offices often. Let them get to know the face of women with heart disease.
- Write advocacy letters or send e-mails to your state legislators, governor, and the U.S. senators and congressional representatives from your district. Tell them about the impact these issues have on women with heart disease. For information on an effective writing campaign, go to http://www.womenheart.org/advocacy.asp.
- Once you've connected with an organization, put yourself in a position where you can talk to the public and the press. Take a public speaking course or one of the advocacy training programs mentioned earlier in this chapter. Do whatever it takes to effectively get the word out. Policy makers will get to know and respect you—and that will help you build your relationship, and keep the issue in the public eye.
- Support the policy makers who support women with heart disease. Make a campaign donation and get other people to do the same.
- Sometimes you can be more effective if you're working with an organization such as the American Heart Association, the Heart Truth Campaign, or WomenHeart. It gives you credibility, resources, and strength. Remember: There's impact in numbers!

Advocacy is very heady stuff! Once I got home I met a lobbyist who directed me to a group of nonprofits known as the Iowa HealthCare Access Network. We started with a lobby day at our state capitol. We were able to hand out our information and talk to our legislators. Letters are frequently written to the editor and I have since been made chairperson of this network. I feel that it is necessary to get the right information to the right people at the right time. I truly feel that I make a difference and that makes me feel good. My heart disease has led me in many directions. The knowledge that I am acquiring gives me a feeling of control in what I at first thought would be a future of feeling out of control.
—Diana, Des Moines, IA, age 55

Take a Stand: The HEART For Women Act

On February 14, 2006, the HEART for Women Act was introduced in Congress. Proposed by a coalition of national health organizations, the bipartisan bill was introduced in the Senate by Senators Debbie Stabenow (D-MI) and Lisa Murkowski (R-AK), and in the House of Representatives by Representatives Lois Capps (D-CA) and Barbara Cubin (R-WY). The HEART for Women Act takes a multipronged approach to improving the prevention, diagnosis, and treatment of heart disease and stroke by proposing to:

- *Raise awareness among women and their health-care providers.* The bill authorizes grants to educate health-care professionals about the prevalence and unique aspects of care for women in the prevention and treatment of cardiovascular diseases. It also authorizes the Medicare program to conduct an educational awareness campaign for older women about their risk for heart disease and stroke.
- *Provide gender- and race-specific information for clinicians and researchers.* The legislation would require that health-care data that is already being reported to the federal government be stratified by gender, as well as by race and ethnicity. Among the information that would be reported by gender includes clinical trial data, pharmaceutical and medical device approval data, medical errors data, hospital quality data, and quality improvement data.
- *Improve screening for low-income women at risk for heart disease and stroke.* The Centers for Disease Control and Prevention (CDC) currently administers a program called WISEWOMAN (Well-Integrated Screening and Evaluation for Women Across the Nation) that provides heart disease and stroke prevention screening, such as tests for high blood pressure and high cholesterol, to low-income uninsured and underinsured women in fourteen states. The legislation would authorize the expansion of WISEWOMAN to all fifty states.

I encourage you to support this vital legislation. This link gives you the information you need to contact your federal legislators regarding the HEART for Women Act: http://www.heartforwomen.org.

Diana is on fire! She got the important training she needed and is in Iowa with a group of women making a difference and enlightening community leaders and policy makers about the needs of women and heart disease. Heart disease puts women in a club they never wanted to belong to, but many women advocates, like Diana, are changing the medical, political, and social system of this country. The seeds are planted—now watch them grow!

Recommended Reading

Books

The African-American Woman's Guide to a Healthy Heart, Anne L. Taylor, MD, Hilton Publishing Company and the Association of Black Cardiologists Center for Women's Health (2004)

Breast Cancer Husband: How to Help Your Wife (and Yourself) Through Diagnosis, Treatment, and Beyond, Marc Silver, Rodale Books (2004)

Building Doctor/Patient Trust, Frank Boehm, MD, Self-published (2006)

Doctors and Their Patients, Edward Shorter, MD, Transaction Publisher (1991)

Fast Food Nation, Eric Schlosser, Houghton Mifflin Company (2001)

Heal Your Heart with Wine and Chocolate, Deborah Yost, Stewart, Tabori and Chang (2006)

The Healthy Heart Handbook for Women, Marian Sandmaier, National Institutes of Health and National Heart, Lung and Blood Institute (2006)

The Heart of the Matter, Hilton M. Hudson II, MD, FACS, and Herbert Stern, PhD, Hilton Publishing Company (2000)

The Heart Speaks: A Cardiologist Reveals the Secret Language of Healing, Mimi Guarneri, MD, FACC, Fusion Press (2006)

Living Through Breast Cancer, Carolyn M. Kaelin, MD, MPH, with Francesca Coltera, McGraw-Hill and Harvard Medical School (2005)

Mayo Clinic Heart Book, Second Edition, Mayo Foundation for Medical Education and Research (2000)

No-Fad Diet, American Heart Association, Clarkson/Potter Publishers (2005)

Nutrition for Women, Elizabeth Somer, MA, RD, Henry Holt and Company (2003)

Satisfaction: Women, Sex, and the Quest for Intimacy, Anita H. Clayton, MD, The Ballantine Publishing Group (2006)

The Savvy Woman Patient, Phyllis Greenberger, MSW, with Jennifer Wider, MD, Capital Books (2006)

Sex and the Seasoned Woman, Gail Sheehy, Random House (2006)

Stories from the Heart: Women Heart Patients Describe Their Disease, Treatment and Recovery, Compiled and arranged by Anastasia Roussos and Melissa Lausin, WomenHeart: The National Coalition for Women with Heart Disease (2003)

Thriving with Heart Disease, Wayne M. Sotile, Ph.D. with Robin Cantor-Cooke, Free Press (2003)

Toxic Friends/True Friends: How Your Friends Can Value or Break Your Health, Happiness, Family and Career, Florence Isaacs, Kensington Publishing Corporation (2003)

What Color is Your Parachute?, Richard Nelson Bolles, Ten Speed Press (2006)

Women are Not Small Men, Nieca Goldberg, MD, Ballantine Publishing Group (2002)

Women Don't Ask, Linda Babcock and Sara Laschever, Princeton University Press (2003)

Magazines

Cooking Light
Web Address: www.cookinglight.com

EatingWell Magazine
Web Address: www.eatingwell.com

Health
Web Address: www.health.com

Healthy Food Guide
Web Address: www.healthyfood.co.nz/

Heart Healthy Living
Web Address: www.hearthealthyonline.com

Prevention
Web Address: www.prevention.com

SELF
Web Address: www.self.com

Shape
Web Address: www.shape.com

Resources

General Information

Agency for Healthcare Research and Quality (AHRQ)
Office of Communications and Knowledge Transfer
540 Gaither Road, Suite 2000
Rockville, MD 20850
Phone: (800) 358-9295
Web Address: http://www.ahcpr.gov
Provides consumer information on the most effective, up-to-date diagnostic and treatment guidelines and research available for many medical conditions including heart disease.

American Association of Retired Persons (AARP)
601 E Street, NW
Washington, DC 20049
Phone: (888) OUR-AARP (888-687-2277)
Web Address: http://www.aarp.org

The American Diabetes Association (ADA)
Phone: (800) DIABETES or (703) 549-1500
Web Address: http://www.diabetes.org
Provides information and resources about the multifaceted issues facing many patients with diabetes.

The American Heart Association
American Heart Association
National Center
7272 Greenville Avenue
Dallas, TX 75231
Phone: (800) AHA-USA-1 or (800) 242-8721
Web Address: http://www.americanheart.org
For Information on CPR:
Phone: (877) AHA-4CPR
Web Address: http://www.americanheart.org/presenter.jhtml?identifier=
3034322.

American Obesity Association
1250 24th Street, NW
Suite 300
Washington, DC 20037
Phone: (202) 776-7711
Fax: (202) 776-7712
Web Address: http://www.obesity.org
The leading organization for education and advocacy on obesity.

The Association of Black Cardiologists Center for Women's Health
Web Address: http://www.abcardio.org
Information about prevention, research, and instructional material
specifically addressing the issues facing African American women with heart
disease.

Dr. Koop
Web Address: http://www.drkoop.com
A medical information site that gives advice on medications and general
health issues.

HeartCenterOnline
Web Address: http://www.heartcenteronline.com
A resource for news and information regarding the heart, such as risk-factor
management and wellness, medications, conditions and procedures, and
treatments and tests. You can sign up to receive their weekly e-newsletters.

Heart Healthy Women
Web address: http://www.hearthealthywomen.org
A source of information for patients and providers for the diagnosis and
treatment of heart disease in women.

Heart Information Network
Web Address: http://www.heartinfo.org
Trustworthy patient information about heart attack, blood pressure,
cholesterol, stroke, diet, and more.

The Heart Truth: A National Awareness Campaign on
Women and Heart Disease
Web Address: http://www.hearttruth.gov or to order a Red Dress Pin
http://emall.nhlbihin.net/product2.asp?sku=56-075N
Provides information about the National Heart, Lung, and Blood Institute's
heart-disease awareness and education campaign for women.

Intelihealth
Web Address: http://www.intelihealth.com/IH/ihtIH/WSIHW000/408/408.htm
A Harvard Medical School consumer-health information site that's
sponsored by Aetna. It gives the reader credible health information from
trusted sources.

Medscape
Web Address: http://www.medscape.com
Detailed medical information on updated research about medical
conditions, including heart disease. You can receive e-newsletters from
them.

National Heart, Lung, and Blood Institute (NHLBI)
Health Information Center
PO Box 30105
Bethesda, MD 20824-0105
Phone: (301) 592-8573
Web Address: http://www.nhlbi.nih.gov
Provides health information for patients, the public, health professionals,
and researchers.
NHLBI Heart Health Information Line
Phone: (800) 575-WELL
Provides toll-free messages with special information for women.

National Women's Health Information Center, Office on Women's Health,
U.S. Department of Health and Human Services
Web Address: http://www.4woman.gov
The federal government's site focusing on general health information for
women.

Society for Women's Health Research
1025 Connecticut Avenue, NW
Suite 710
Washington, DC 20036
Phone: (202) 223-8224
Web Address: http://www.womenshealthresearch.org/site/PageServer

WebMD
Web Address: http://www.webmd.com
A source of information for many medical conditions, including heart
disease. You can get their weekly e-newsletter with updated medical
research on diagnostic procedures and treatments, as well as recent news
about heart disease.

WomenHeart: The National Coalition for Women with Heart Disease
818 18th Street, NW
Suite 930
Washington, DC 20006
Phone: (202) 728-7199
Web Address: http://www.womenheart.org

The Women's Health Site
Web Address: http://www.thewomenshealthsite.org/01_home/index.jsp
A Duke University Medical Center Web site designed for health-care
professionals, it features information about new developments in women's
health care.

Mental Health, Marriage, and Family

American Association for Marriage and Family Therapy
112 South Alfred Street
Alexandria, VA 22314-3061
Phone: (703) 839-9808
Web Address: http://www.aamft.org/index_nm.asp
Source for a referral to a qualified family therapist near you.

American Association of Pastoral Counselors
9504A Lee Highway
Fairfax, VA 22031-2303
Phone: (703) 385-6967
Fax: (703) 352-7725
Email: info@aapc.org
Web Address: http://www.aapc.org
A referral source to find certified pastoral counselors in your area.

American Psychiatric Association
1000 Wilson Boulevard, Suite 1825
Arlington, VA 22209-3901
Phone: (703) 907-7300 or (888) 357-7924
Email: apa@psych.org
Web Address: http://www.psych.org
Contact them for a referral to a psychiatrist in your area.

American Psychological Association
750 First Street, NE
Washington, DC 20002-4242
Phone: (800) 374-2721 or (202) 336-5500; TDD/TTY: (202) 336-6123
For a referral to a clinical psychologist: (800) 964-2000
Web Address: http://www.apa.org

American Self-Help Group Clearinghouse
Phone: (973) 326-6789
Web Address: http://www.selfhelpgroups.org
A large database for finding self-help groups near you.

Anxiety Disorders Association of America
8730 Georgia Avenue, Suite 600
Silver Spring, MD 20910
Phone: (240) 485-1001
Web Address: http://www.adaa.org

The Coalition for Marriage, Family & Couples Education
5310 Belt Road, NW
Washington, DC 20015-1961
Phone: (202) 362-3332
Web Address: http://www.smartmarriages.com
A resource for information exchange and to help couples locate marriage
and relationship courses.

Depression and Bipolar Support Network
730 N. Franklin Street, Suite 501
Chicago, Illinois 60610-7224
Phone: (312) 642-0049 or (800) 826-3632
Fax: (312) 642-7243
Web Address: http://www.dbsalliance.org

The Mended Hearts, Inc. (Affiliated with the American Heart Association)
7272 Greenville Avenue
Dallas, TX 75231-4596
Phone: (888) HEART99 or (888) 432-7899
Email: info@mendedhearts.org
Web Address: http://www.mendedhearts.org
They offer support groups nationally to patients who have had a heart
event, and can refer you to a support group in your area.

National Institute of Mental Health
Phone: (301) 443-4513
Web Address: http://www.nimh.nih.gov

National Mental Health Association
Phone: (800) 969-6642
Web Address: http://www.nmha.org

WomenHeart: The National Coalition for Women with Heart Disease
Phone: (202) 728-7199
Web Address (English): http://www.womenheart.org
Web Address (Spanish): http://www.espanol.womenheart.org
Information on locations of support networks across the country.

CAREGIVER SUPPORT

Caregiving.com
Web Address: http://www.caregiving.com
Provides an online support network for caregivers.

Family Caregiver Alliance (FCA)
180 Montgomery Street, Suite 1100
San Francisco, CA 94104
Phone: (415) 434-3388 or (800) 445-8106
Email: info@caregiver.org
Web Address: http://www.caregiver.org

Heartmates
Phone: (612) 558-3331
Web Address: http://www.heartmates.com
Spouse, family, or friends of heart patients can receive online support and
comfort. Heartmates also offers updated information for caregivers.

National Organization for Empowering Caregivers
Web Address: http://www.nofec.org and http://www.care-givers.com
A resource list, newsletter, chat area, featured expert guests and more.

Body Image and the Sexual Self

American Association of Sex Educators, Counselors, and Therapists
P.O. Box 5488
Richmond, VA 23220-0488
Phone: (319) 895-8407
Web Address: http://www.aasect.org

The American Board of Sexology
Web Address: http://www.sexologist.org

The Hypnosis Network
Web Address: http://www.hypnosisnetwork.com

Medline Plus
Web Address: http://www.nlm.nih.gov/medlineplus/ency/article/001487.htm

National Foundation for Sexual Health Medicine
Web Address: http://www.nfshm.org

North American Menopause Society
Web Address: http://www.menopause.org

Career Information and Rights

The American Heart Association
Web Address: http://post.americanheart.org/haw
Information on how to raise awareness at work.

Employment Opportunity Commission
Web Address: http://www.eeoc.gov or
http://www.eeoc.gov/policy/docs/preemp.html

National Career Development Association
Web Address: http://www.ncda.org

U.S. Department of Labor, Office of Disability Employment Policy
Web Address: http://www.dol.gov/odep/archives/ek96/inquiry.htm

NUTRITION, EXERCISE, AND RISK-FACTOR REDUCTION

Weight Control and Diet

Activity Calorie Counter
Web Address: http://www.primusweb.com/fitnesspartner/jumpsite/calculat.htm
Tells you how many calories you burn in comparison to the calories you
consume.

American Association of Nutritional Sciences
Web Address: http://www.nutrition.org
For Recent Publications: http://pubs.nutrition.org

American Dietetic Association
216 West Jackson Blvd.
Chicago, IL 60606-6995
Phone: (312) 899-0040
Web Address: http://www.eatright.org
Focuses on nutrition, health, and well-being.

American Heart Association (AHA)
Food Pyramid Information:
Web Addresses:
Food Pyramid Information: http://www.deliciousdecisions.org/ee/afp.html.
AHA publications: http://www.ahajournals.org/

Calorie Control Council
Web Address: http://www.caloriecontrol.org
Helpful information for cutting calories and fat in your diet, and achieving
and maintaining a healthy weight. It also provide tips on low-calorie,
reduced-fat foods and beverages.

Choose to Lose
Web Address: http://www.choicediets.com
Offers weight-loss and cholesterol-lowering programs, and books to help
people reach their ideal weight and lower their cholesterol in a healthy way.

CyberDiet
Web Address: http://www.cyberdiet.com
A commercial online weight-loss program.

eDiets
Web Address: http://www.dietcity.com
A commercial online weight-loss program.

Harvard School of Public Health
Department of Nutrition
665 Huntington Avenue
Boston, MA 02115
Phone: (617) 432-1851
Web Address: http://www.hsph.harvard.edu/nutritionsource
This Web site helps people get on the healthiest diet available by exploring
the most recent research about healthy eating habits.

Healthy Dining Finder
Web Address: http://www.HealthyDiningFinder.com
A heart-healthy restaurant locator for the entire country.
Phone: (800) 953-DINE(3463)

The Hypnosis Network
Web Address: http://www.hypnosisnetwork.com
Designed to help women successfully implement their own healthy eating
and weight-loss program.

Mayo Clinic's Food and Nutrition Center
Web Address: http://www.mayoclinic.com/findinformation/conditioncenters
/centers.cfm?objectid=000851DA-6222-1B37-8D7E80C8D77A0000
This site is designed to help people find out about food and nutrition by
exploring what constitutes a healthy diet, including healthy cooking and eating.

National Heart, Lung, and Blood Institute (NHLBI)
PO Box 7923
Bethesda, MD 20824-0104
Phone: (301) 592-8573
Web Addresses:
Calculate Your Body Mass Index: http://www.nhlbisupport.com/bmi.
Classifications of Being Overweight or Obese: http://www.nhlbi.nih.gov
/health/public/heart/obesity/lose_wt/bmi_dis.htm
Healthy Weight: http://www.nhlbi.nih.gov/health/public/heart/obesity
/lose_wt/index.htm
Heart Healthy Recipes: http://www.nhlbi.nih.gov/health/public/heart/
other/syah/index.htm

National Institutes of Health
Web Address: http://hp2010.nhlbihin.net/portion
This site gives you a quiz on what your portion distortions are when you eat.

Nutrition Data Analyzer
Web Address: http://www.nutritiondata.com
Analyzes all the nutrients in the foods or recipes you eat and will guide you to eat the foods that have the best dietary value for you.

Take Pounds Off Sensibly (TOPS)
Web Address: http://www.tops.org
Offers fellowship, caring, and a supportive approach to weight loss and control.

Weight Watchers
Web Address: http://www.weightwatchers.com/index.aspx
By clicking on this site you can find a Weight Watchers near you. Weight Watchers is a commercial weight-loss program.

Fitness Options

American Association of Cardiovascular and Pulmonary Rehabilitation
401 North Michigan Avenue
Suite 2200
Chicago, IL 60622-4267
Phone: (312) 321-5146
Web Address: http://www.aacvpr.org
The association's goal is to promote health and prevent disease through cardiac rehabilitation.

American Council on Exercise (ACE)
Web Address: http://www.acefitness.org
The goal of this organization is to enrich the quality of lives through safe and effective physical activity.

Kathy Smith, "Your Leader in Total Fitness"
Web Address: http://www.kathysmith.com

Melpomene Institute
Web Address: http://www.melpomene.org
Helps girls and women of all ages understand the link between physical activity and health through research, publications, and education.

The National Institute for Fitness and Sport (NIFS)
Web Address: http://www.nifs.org
The goal of this organization is to enhance health, physical fitness, and athletic performance through research, education, and service.

Shape Up America!
Web Address: http://www.shapeup.org
Offers tips and programs to help you manage your weight, improve your fitness, and learn healthy eating habits.

YWCA of the USA
Web Address: http://www.ywca.org
The goal of this organization is to eliminate racism and empower women through advocacy, education, training, and physical fitness.

Other National Heart, Lung, and Blood Institute Sites for Risk Factor Reduction

For Blood Pressure: http://www.nhlbi.nih.gov/hbp/index.html

What You Need to Know about Having High Cholesterol:
http://www.nhlbi.nih.gov/health/public/heart/chol/hbc_what.htm

Lowering Cholesterol: http://www.nhlbi.nih.gov/chd

Heart Attack Signs: http://www.nhlbi.nih.gov/actintime/index.htm

Smoking-cessation Information

American Cancer Society
1599 Clifton Road, NE
Atlanta, GA 30329-4251
Phone: (800) 227-2345
Web Address: http://www.cancer.org

American Lung Association
61 Broadway, 6th Floor
New York, NY 10006
Phone: (800) 586-4872, (212) 315-8700 and to speak to a lung health professional call (800) 548-8252
Web Address: http://www.lungusa.org
The ALA can refer you to a local chapter near you.

Medication Management

American Society of Health-System Pharmacists
7272 Wisconsin Avenue
Bethesda, MD 20814
Phone: (301) 657-3000
Web Address: http://www.safemedication.com
Provides patients with information about the medications that they're taking
and any potential side effects so that they can determine whether they're
taking effective and safe medications.

Benefits Check Up Rx
Web Address: http://www.benefitscheckup.org
A service of the National Council on Aging that helps people connect to
private or government programs to help pay for prescription drugs, health
care, utilities, and other needs.

Center Watch
Web Address: http://www.centerwatch.com
Provides information regarding more than 41,000 active industry- and
government-sponsored clinical trials and new drug therapies in research
and those recently approved by the FDA.

Drug Store
Web Address: http://drugstore.com
You can fill new prescriptions and get refills through this leading online
pharmacy. This site has a pharmacist on duty twenty-four hours per day, and if
there are potential harmful drug interactions, the pharmacist will contact you.

Food and Drug Administration (FDA)
Web Address: http://www.fda.gov/womens/tttc.html
This is a national campaign sponsored by the FDA's Office of Women's
Health, which aims to educate women about the safe use of medication.

National Pharmaceutical Council
Web Address: http://yourpharmacybenefit.org/
Explains some of the terminology and the process of insurance plans in
general.

Partnership for Prescription Assistance (PPARx)
Phone: (888) 477-2669
Web Address: http://www.pparx.org/Intro.php
This program helps qualifying patients who lack prescription coverage get
their prescription medications paid for through private or public programs.

Rx List
Web Address: http://www.rxlist.com
Gives consumers and professionals information about prescription
medications, their side effects, clinical trials, and dosages.

Rx.com
Web Address: http://www.rx.com
A leading online pharmacy.

Hospitals and Health-care Providers

American Board of Medical Specialties
1007 Church St, Suite 404
Evanston, IL 60201-5913
Phone: (866) 275-2267
Web Address: http://www.abms.org
This organization represent twenty-four medical specialty boards and
establishes high standards for medical certification in a doctor's field of
specialty. ABMS has the goal of insuring high-quality and safe medical
service by a certified medical specialist. This is a site you can use to make
sure your specialist is certified in his/her medical specialty.

American Heart Association
Web Address: http://216.185.112.5/presenter.jhtml?identifier=4678
Has a list of questions you can ask your doctor.

The Best Heart Hospitals List—Recommended by WomenHeart
Web Address: http://www.womenheart.org/information/
access_to_healthcare.asp#best

Hospital Accreditation
Joint Commission on Accreditation of Healthcare Organizations
One Renaissance Boulevard
Oakbrook Terrace, IL 60181
Phone: (708) 916-5600
Web Address: http://www.jcaho.org

U.S. Department of Health and Human Services
Web Address: http://www.hospitalcompare.hhs.gov
This site gives consumers a tool to compare how different hospitals in your
area deliver care to adult patients.

WomenHeart Support Network Locations
Web Address: http://www.womenheart.org/city_support_network.asp

Women's Heart Centers
Web Address: http://www.womenheart.org/home_resources/resources_1.asp

Health Plan Information

American Association of Retired Persons (AARP) Health Care Options
Web Address: http://www.aarphealthcare.com
If you're having problems with your managed care plan, this is a good place
to go for information.

Best's Insurance Resources
State Regulatory Agencies
Web Address: http://www.ambest.com/directory/govdir.html?l=1&Menu=
Industry+Resources,State+Insurance+Regulators
This site will help you find insurance regulatory agencies in your area.

Consumers' Groups

American Medical Consumers
5415 Briggs Avenue
La Crescenta, CA 91214
Phone: (818) 957-3508
Web Address: http://www.medconsumer.com

Consumer Coalition for Quality Health Care
1101 Vermont Avenue, NW, Suite 1001
Washington, DC 20005
Phone: (202) 789-3606
Fax: (202) 898-2389
Web Address: http://www.consumers.org

Consumers' Union
101 Truman Avenue
Yonkers, NY 10703
Phone: (914) 378-2000

Health Insurance Consumer Information
Web Address: http://www.quotit.net/resources/terms_health2.htm
Gives the reader consumer information on various types of insurance plans.

Health Plan Accreditation
National Committee for Quality Assurance
2000 L Street, NW
Suite 500

Washington, DC 20036
Phone: (202) 955-3500
Web Address: http://www.ncqa.org

Health Savings Account Information (HSA)
Web Address: http://www.treasury.gov/offices/public-affairs/hsa

Insure.com
Web Address: http://info.insure.com/health/hipaa.html
Gives the reader information on HIPAA.

Medicare
Phone: (800) Medicare
Web Address: http://www.medicare.gov

National Association of Insurance Commissioners
Web Address: http://www.naic.org/state_web_map.htm
This is a site that will help you find an insurance commissioner in your area.

Patient Advocacy Foundation
700 Thimble Shoals Boulevard, Suite 200
Newport News, VA 23606
Phone: (800) 532-5274
Fax: (757) 873-8999
E-Mail: help@patientadvocate.org
Web Address: http://www.patientadvocate.org
This organization can help advocate on your behalf regarding health insurance issues.

HEALTH CARE RIGHTS AND RESPONSIBILITIES

President's Advisory Commission on Consumer Protection & Quality in the Health Care Industry
Web Address: http://www.hcqualitycommission.gov/final/append_a.html
The Quality Interagency Coordination Task Force
Patients Rights and Responsibilities
Web Address: http://www.consumer.gov/qualityhealth/rights.htm.

DISABILITY INFORMATION

Social Security Administration
Phone: (800) 772-1213
Web Address: http://www.ssa.gov or www.socialsecurity.gov

International Organizations

Australia

Australian Women's Health Network
64 Pennington Tce
North Adelaide
South Australia
Australia 5006
Phone: 08 8239 9644
Web Address: http://www.awhn.org.au

Cardiac Society of Australia and New Zealand (CSANZ)
145 Macquarie Street
Sydney, NSW 2000
Australia
Phone: +61 2 9256 5452
Email: info@csanz.edu.au
Web Address: http://www.medeserv.com.au/csanz

Diabetes Australia
GPO BOX 3156
Canberra ACT 2601
Help line: 1300 136 588
Phone: 02 6232 3800
Web Address: http://www.diabetesaustralia.com.au

HealthInsite
HealthInsite Section
Department of Health and Ageing, MDP 2
GPO Box 9848
Canberra ACT 2601
Phone: 02 6289 8488
Web Address: http://www.healthinsite.gov.au

Heart Foundation
(Australian Capital Territory Division)
15 Denison St.
Deakin ACT 2600
Phone: 02 6282 5744
Heartline: 1300 36 27 87
Web Address: http://www.heartfoundation.com.au

Heart Support—Australia
Unit 7b 52 Wollongong Street
Fyshwick ACT 2609
Phone: 02 6280 7211
Web Address: http://www.heartnet.org.au

National Heart Foundation (Australian Capital Territory Division)
15 Denison Street
Deakin ACT 2600
Phone: 02 6282 5744
Heartline: 13300 36 27 87
Web Address: http://www.heartfoundation.com.au

New Zealand

Cardiac Society of Australia and New Zealand (CSANZ)
145 Macquarie Street
Sydney, NSW 2000
Australia
Phone: +61 2 9256 5452
Email: info@csanz.edu.au
Web Address: http://www.medeserv.com.au/csanz

Diabetes New Zealand
PO Box 12-441
Thorndon, Wellington
New Zealand
Phone: 0800 DIABETES
Email: info@diabetes.org.nz
Web Address: http://www.diabetes.org.nz

Ministry of Health
Phone: 0800 611 116
Web Address: http://www.moh.govt.nz

The National Heart Foundation of New Zealand
PO Box 17-160, Greenlane
9 Kalmia Street, Ellerslie
Auckland 1130
New Zealand
Phone: +64 09 571 9191
Email: info@nhf.org.nz
Web Address: http://www.nhf.org.nz

Women's Health Action
PO Box 9947
Newmarket, Auckland
New Zealand
Phone: +64 9 520 5295
Web Address: http://www.womens-health.org.nz

United Kingdom

Big Matters
Web Address: http://www.bigmatters.co.uk
Obesity support community.

British Cardiac Patients Association
2 Station Road
Swavesey, Cambridge CB4 5QJ
Phone: 0800 4792800
Web Address: http://www.bcpa.co.uk
Help and support for cardiac patients and their families.

British Heart Foundation
14 Fitzhardinge Street
London W1H 6DH
Phone: 020 7935 0185
Web Address: http://www.bhf.org.uk

Department of Health
Richmond House
79 Whitehall
London SW1A 2NS
Phone: 020 7210 5025
Web Address: http://www.dh.gov.uk
New articles on a variety of health topics and general health information.

Diabetes UK
Macleod House,
10 Parkway, London NW1 7AA
Phone: 020 7424 1000
Web Address: http://www.diabetes.org.uk

Healthy Heart Programme
Web Address: http://www.heartpro.co.uk

Heyday
Web Address: http://www.heyday.org.uk
UK organization for retired people.

Women's Health Concern
Health Concern Ltd.
Whitehall House
41 Whitehall
London
SW1A 2BY
Phone: 020 7451 1377
Web Address: http://www.womens-health-concern.org
Women's health information.

ACKNOWLEDGMENTS

My heartfelt thanks to all the women heart patient survivors and their families in this country. And to the ones who lost their battle to heart disease—your voices and your messages echo throughout the book and will be a guide and support to others. Forever we're "Heart Sisters."

Thanks to everyone involved with WomenHeart: The National Coalition for Women with Heart Disease, especially the inspirational board of directors, advisory board, and fabulous staff. To Nancy Loving and Dr. Sharonne Hayes, you're the ones who listened and gave me my life back. I will be forever grateful. Your constant support, advice, and guidance gave me the incentive to keep moving in the right direction with the project.

I am very grateful to the Heart Truth Campaign team of the National Heart, Lung, and Blood Institute. Terry Long, Dr. Ann Taubenheim, and Dr. Elizabeth Nabel have encouraged and supported this project since the beginning. Your help with the message and the statistics were invaluable and important—you helped give the book substance and validity.

I'm indebted to Rhoda Baer, the award-winning photographer who took the white blouse photo and many others including the Real Women photograph for the Heart Truth Campaign. Everyone asks how I was so relaxed ". . . doing a photo like that where you're kind of undressed?" I told them that all you have to do is send a woman away from her husband and kids, give her a makeup stylist and hairdresser, a glass of wine, take her underwear off, have her open her blouse and blow a fan at her. Then have Rhoda and others fuss over her and make her laugh and then *voila,* you get a fabulous picture. But actually Rhoda is an artistic talent bar none. She's the greatest.

Nanette Wenger, MD is one of my heroes and a mentor. She's considered the mother of women's cardiology and has devoted her life to the cause. Dr. Wenger has been a fabulous resource to me, and has given me tremendous encouragement and support. From the bottom of my heart, I appreciate all you do.

A special and gracious thanks to the top doctors and health-care professionals in the country who helped me on this project: Noel Bairey-Merz, MD, Susan Bennett, MD, Kathy Berra, MSN/ANP, Anita Clayton, MD, Senate Majority Leader Bill Frist (MD), Phillip J. Goldstein, MD, Sharonne Hayes, MD, Carolyn Kaelin, MD, MPH, Michael B. Kastan, MD, PhD, Kimberly Kiddoo, PhD, Penny Kris-Etherton, PhD, RD, Jennifer Mieres, MD, Elizabeth Nabel, MD, Clay Semenkovich, MD, Shashana Shiloh, PhD, Stacy Smith, MD, Wayne Sotile, PhD, Ann Taubenheim, PhD, and Nanette K. Wenger, MD. I'm eternally grateful for all you do for all of us.

Sometimes life just puts you in places where you get to meet the most terrific human beings. My thanks and gratitude go out to the following contributors: The American Heart Association's Southeast Affiliate, Robin Cantor-Cooke, John Capecci, Cigna Corporation, Angie Davis, JD, Ed Faruolo, Tommy Gerber, JD, NCCPT, Gary Goldstein, John Goldstein, Howard Green, Phyllis Greenberger, Kathleen Hopper, Joanne Howes, Nathan James, Ted Libernini, Lyn Lindsay, Terry Long, Nancy Loving, Dexter Nash, Kathy Smith (Your Leader in Total Fitness), Society for Women's Health Research, Jill Steinberg, JD, Ken Steinberg, James Tissot and Bette Walters, JD, Emily Yellin, and Debora Yost.

The words "thank you" just aren't good enough for my friend and colleague, writer and editor Susan Dynerman, who is a published author herself. Her experience was invaluable in getting this project off the ground and her writing skills gave the book energy, clarity, and depth. Susan gave me guidance and direction when I'd get lost in the work. I couldn't have done it without her. Susan, you know I think you're awesome.

Joelle Delbourgo is the best agent in the world. Every detail of her work is done with style, professionalism, and a true devotion to the project. She took care of me, was patient and kind, timely, and always thought about the meaning behind this project in every move she made. Thanks for everything.

A tremendous thanks go out to Marnie Cochran of Da Capo Lifelong Books. She's the greatest. I feel so lucky to have her working with me on this project. She also "gets it"—the meaning and importance of the work. Marnie is always timely, communicative, thoughtful, and patient. Her editing skills and marketing prowess are unmatched anywhere.

I am truly grateful to the entire staff of DaCapo Lifelong Books, who have actively been supporting this project with their hearts and souls. Your hard work furthers the cause and is greatly appreciated.

My friends, who are scattered like the wind in California, Maryland, Missouri, North Carolina, New York, Tennessee, Virginia, and Israel: You're simply the greatest people to be with and to know. You inspire me while simultaneously grounding me in what's important. One of my favorite sayings is simple: Love is a verb. You show that reciprocal love—it's unending. Thanks for always being there.

My greatest thanks to Mildred and Sammie Hardin and to Diane and Booker Morris: Without you things would never get done and life just wouldn't be the same. All of you are like family to me.

To my extended family near and far, who are there for me in thick and thin. You gave me feedback and encouragement that was invaluable. Some of you even read the book in the very preliminary stages but your excitement helped me to carry on. And to Doris Kastan, my mother-in-law, who told me, "The book makes me feel like you're holding my hand." Thanks to all of you for all your love!

And thanks especially to my dad who always knows when I need a hug and more than that who gave me the most magical and best-tasting soda and oranges while I was recovering in the hospital.

And bittersweet thanks to my mom and grandma, who succumbed to heart disease—together we were a triumvirate. You lived your lives with grace, strength, and tremendous love—you helped shape the woman I've become. You'll always be on my shoulder coaching me forward—your spirit and determination will always be a part of me.

INDEX

ABOUT THE RED DRESS

Created in 2002 by The Heart Truth—a national awareness campaign sponsored by the federal government's National Heart, Lung, and Blood Institute—the Red Dress was launched as the national symbol for women and heart disease awareness at New York's Fashion Week in February 2003. Coupled with the slogan, "Heart Disease Doesn't Care What You Wear—It's the #1 Killer of Women," the Red Dress is a red alert that inspires women to take action to protect their heart health. The Red Dress has sparked a national movement that is being embraced by millions who share the common goal of greater awareness and heart health for all women.